Undergoing gallbladder surgery is a significant step toward better health for many, yet it comes with its own set of challenges, particularly when it comes to adjusting your diet. The gallbladder plays a crucial role in digesting fats, and its absence requires a thoughtful approach to eating that supports sensitive digestion and reduces inflammation.

"No Gallbladder Diet Cookbook: Eating Well After Surgery" is your essential guide to navigating the dietary adjustments necessary post-surgery. This book is meticulously crafted to help you transition smoothly into a new eating routine, ensuring that your body receives the nutrition it needs while minimizing discomfort and promoting healing.

Inside, you'll find a comprehensive 100-day meal plan designed with over 100 recipes tailored specifically for those without a gallbladder. Each recipe focuses on ingredients that are easy to digest, anti-inflammatory, and nutrient-dense. From breakfast to dinner, and everything in between, this cookbook offers a variety of delicious and healthy options that cater to your new dietary needs.

This cookbook is more than just a collection of recipes; it's a supportive companion on your journey to recovery. You'll discover tips on managing common post-surgery symptoms, advice on portion sizes, and insights into foods that can aid digestion. With clear instructions and helpful nutritional information, each recipe is designed to make meal preparation simple and enjoyable.

Whether you are newly recovering from surgery or looking to maintain a balanced diet without a gallbladder, ***"No Gallbladder Diet Cookbook"*** empowers you to take control of your health through mindful eating. Let's embark on this journey together, transforming your meals into a source of healing and vitality.

I. Grilled chicken breast with steamed broccoli

Ingredient:

• 2 boneless, skinless chicken breasts
• Salt and pepper to taste
• 1 tablespoon olive oil
• 2 cups broccoli florets
• Lemon wedges for serving

Instructions:

1. Preheat your grill to medium·high heat.

2. Season the chicken breasts with salt, pepper, and olive oil.

3. Grill the chicken breasts for about 6·7 minutes per side, or until they are cooked through and reach an internal temperature of 165°F (74°C).

4. While the chicken is grilling, steam the broccoli florets until they are tender but still crisp, about 5·7 minutes.

5. Serve the grilled chicken breasts with the steamed broccoli on the side. Squeeze some fresh lemon juice over the chicken before serving for extra flavor.

This meal is low in fat and easy to digest, making it a good choice for those following a no gallbladder diet. Enjoy!

2. Baked salmon with dill and lemon

Ingredient:

- 2 salmon fillets
- Salt and pepper to taste
- 2 tablespoons olive oil
- 2 tablespoons fresh dill, chopped
- 1 lemon, sliced
- 2 cloves garlic, minced

Instructions:

1. Preheat your oven to 375°F (190°C).

2. Season the salmon fillets with salt and pepper on both sides.

3. Place the salmon fillets on a baking sheet lined with parchment paper.

4. Drizzle the olive oil over the salmon fillets.

5. Sprinkle the chopped dill and minced garlic over the salmon.

6. Place lemon slices on top of the salmon fillets.

7. Bake in the preheated oven for about 15•20 minutes, or until the salmon is cooked through and flakes easily with a fork.

8. Serve the baked salmon with dill and lemon alongside your favorite side dishes.

This dish is rich in omega•3 fatty acids and is gentle on the digestive system, making it a great option for a no gallbladder diet. Enjoy your meal!

3. Turkey meatballs with marinara sauce

Ingredient:

For the turkey meatballs:
• 1 pound ground turkey
• 1/2 cup breadcrumbs
• 1/4 cup grated Parmesan cheese
• 1 egg
• 2 cloves garlic, minced
• 1 teaspoon dried oregano
• Salt and pepper to taste
• 2 tablespoons olive oil

For the marinara sauce:
• 1 can (14 oz) crushed tomatoes
• 2 cloves garlic, minced
• 1 teaspoon dried basil
• 1 teaspoon dried oregano
• Salt and pepper to taste

Instructions:
1. Preheat your oven to 400°F (200°C).

2. In a mixing bowl, combine the ground turkey, breadcrumbs, Parmesan cheese, egg, minced garlic, dried oregano, salt, and pepper. Mix until well combined.

3. Shape the mixture into meatballs of your desired size.

4. Heat olive oil in a skillet over medium heat. Brown the meatballs on all sides, then transfer them to a baking dish.

5. In the same skillet, add crushed tomatoes, minced garlic, dried basil, dried oregano, salt, and pepper. Simmer for a few minutes to combine the flavors.

6. Pour the marinara sauce over the meatballs in the baking dish.

7. Bake in the preheated oven for about 20•25 minutes, or until the meatballs are cooked through.

8. Serve the turkey meatballs with marinara sauce over pasta or zucchini noodles, if desired.

4. Quinoa salad with cucumber and cherry tomatoes

Ingredient:

• 1 cup quinoa
• 2 cups water or vegetable broth
• 1 cucumber, diced
• 1 cup cherry tomatoes, halved
• 1/4 cup red onion, finely chopped
• 1/4 cup fresh parsley, chopped
• 1/4 cup feta cheese, crumbled (optional)
• Juice of 1 lemon
• 2 tablespoons olive oil
• Salt and pepper to taste

Instructions:

1. Rinse the quinoa under cold water. In a saucepan, combine the quinoa and water or vegetable broth. Bring to a boil, then reduce heat, cover, and simmer for about 15 minutes, or until the quinoa is cooked and the liquid is absorbed. Fluff with a fork and let it cool.

2. In a large bowl, combine the cooked quinoa, diced cucumber, cherry tomatoes, red onion, and parsley.

3. In a small bowl, whisk together the lemon juice, olive oil, salt, and pepper.

4. Pour the dressing over the quinoa salad and toss to combine.

5. If using, sprinkle the crumbled feta cheese on top.

6. Chill the salad in the refrigerator for about 30 minutes before serving to allow the flavors to meld together.

This quinoa salad is packed with protein, fiber, and vitamins, making it a healthy and gallbladder•friendly option. Enjoy this light and flavorful dish!

5. Lentil soup with carrots and celery

Ingredient:

• 1 cup dried lentils, rinsed and drained
• 4 cups vegetable broth
• 1 onion, chopped
• 2 carrots, diced
• 2 celery stalks, diced
• 2 cloves garlic, minced
• 1 teaspoon dried thyme
• 1 teaspoon dried oregano
• Salt and pepper to taste
• 2 tablespoons olive oil
• Fresh parsley for garnish

Instructions:

1. In a large pot, heat olive oil over medium heat. Add the chopped onion, carrots, celery, and garlic. Cook until the vegetables are softened, about 5•7 minutes.

2. Add the dried lentils, vegetable broth, dried thyme, dried oregano, salt, and pepper to the pot. Bring to a boil, then reduce heat and simmer for about 20•25 minutes, or until the lentils are tender.

3. Using an immersion blender, partially blend the soup to thicken it while still leaving some lentils whole for texture. Alternatively, you can blend a portion of the soup in a blender and return it to the pot.

4. Adjust seasoning with salt and pepper if needed.

5. Serve the lentil soup hot, garnished with fresh parsley.

This lentil soup is high in fiber, protein, and nutrients, making it a healthy and gallbladder•friendly choice. Enjoy this hearty and delicious soup!

6. Vegetable stir•fry with tofu or lean beef

Ingredient:

• 1 block of firm tofu, drained and cubed OR 1/2 pound lean beef, thinly sliced
• 2 tablespoons soy sauce
• 1 tablespoon sesame oil
• 1 tablespoon cornstarch
• 1 tablespoon vegetable oil
• 2 cloves garlic, minced
• 1 inch piece of ginger, grated
• Assorted vegetables (such as bell peppers, broccoli, carrots, snap peas)
• Salt and pepper to taste
• Cooked rice or quinoa for serving

Instructions:

1. If using tofu, marinate the cubed tofu in soy sauce, sesame oil, and cornstarch for about 15•20 minutes. If using beef, marinate the sliced beef in the same mixture.

2. Heat vegetable oil in a large skillet or wok over medium•high heat. Add the minced garlic and grated ginger, and sauté for about 1 minute until fragrant.

3. Add the marinated tofu or beef to the skillet and cook until browned and cooked through.

4. Add the assorted vegetables to the skillet and stir•fry until they are tender•crisp.

5. Season with salt and pepper to taste.

6. Serve the vegetable stir•fry with tofu or lean beef over cooked rice or quinoa.

This dish is high in protein and fiber, and the vegetables provide essential nutrients, making it a healthy and gallbladder•friendly meal option. Enjoy this flavorful and satisfying stir•fry!

7. Egg white omelette with spinach and mushrooms

Ingredient:

• 4 egg whites
• 1 cup fresh spinach, chopped
• 1/2 cup mushrooms, sliced
• 1/4 cup onion, chopped
• Salt and pepper to taste
• 1 teaspoon olive oil

Instructions:

1. In a bowl, whisk the egg whites until frothy. Season with salt and pepper.

2. Heat olive oil in a non•stick skillet over medium heat.

3. Add the chopped onion and sliced mushrooms to the skillet and sauté until softened.

4. Add the chopped spinach to the skillet and cook until wilted.

5. Pour the whisked egg whites over the vegetables in the skillet.

6. Cook the omelette, lifting the edges with a spatula to let the uncooked egg flow underneath.

7. Once the egg is set, fold the omelette in half and cook for another minute.

8. Slide the omelette onto a plate and serve hot.

This egg white omelette with spinach and mushrooms is high in protein and low in fat, making it a healthy and gallbladder•friendly breakfast or meal option. Enjoy this light and flavorful omelette!

8. Grilled shrimp skewers with bell peppers

Ingredient:

• 1 pound large shrimp, peeled and deveined
• 1 red bell pepper, cut into chunks
• 1 yellow bell pepper, cut into chunks
• 1 green bell pepper, cut into chunks
• 2 tablespoons olive oil
• 2 cloves garlic, minced
• 1 teaspoon paprika
• Salt and pepper to taste
• Wooden skewers, soaked in water

Instructions:

1. In a bowl, combine the olive oil, minced garlic, paprika, salt, and pepper.

2. Add the shrimp to the bowl and toss to coat evenly. Marinate for about 15•20 minutes.
3. Preheat the grill to medium•high heat.

4. Thread the marinated shrimp and bell pepper chunks onto the soaked wooden skewers, alternating between shrimp and peppers.

5. Grill the skewers for about 2•3 minutes per side, or until the shrimp are pink and opaque.

6. Remove the skewers from the grill and serve hot.

This grilled shrimp skewers with bell peppers dish is low in fat and high in protein, making it a healthy and gallbladder•friendly option. Enjoy these flavorful and colorful skewers as a light and satisfying meal!

9. Baked cod with roasted asparagus

Ingredient:

• 2 cod fillets
• 1 bunch of asparagus, trimmed
• 2 tablespoons olive oil
• 2 cloves garlic, minced
• 1 lemon, sliced
• Salt and pepper to taste
• Fresh parsley for garnish

Instructions:

1. Preheat your oven to 400°F (200°C).

2. Place the trimmed asparagus on a baking sheet and drizzle with 1 tablespoon of olive oil. Season with salt and pepper.

3. In a small bowl, mix the minced garlic with the remaining olive oil.

4. Place the cod fillets on the baking sheet with the asparagus. Brush the cod fillets with the garlic•infused olive oil.

5. Place lemon slices on top of the cod fillets.

6. Bake in the preheated oven for about 15•20 minutes, or until the cod is cooked through and flakes easily with a fork.

7. Serve the baked cod with roasted asparagus hot, garnished with fresh parsley.

This baked cod with roasted asparagus dish is low in fat and high in protein, making it a healthy and gallbladder•friendly option. Enjoy this simple and delicious meal!

10. Greek yogurt with honey and berries

Ingredient:

• 1 cup Greek yogurt
• 1 tablespoon honey
• Assorted berries (such as strawberries, blueberries, raspberries)
• Optional toppings: chopped nuts, granola, or chia seeds

Instructions:

1. In a bowl, spoon the Greek yogurt.

2. Drizzle the honey over the yogurt.

3. Top the yogurt with assorted berries.

4. Add any optional toppings you desire, such as chopped nuts, granola, or chia seeds.

II. Zucchini noodles with marinara sauce

Ingredient:

• 2•3 medium zucchinis
• 1 cup marinara sauce
• 1 tablespoon olive oil
• 2 cloves garlic, minced
• Salt and pepper to taste
• Grated Parmesan cheese for garnish (optional)
• Fresh basil leaves for garnish

Instructions:

1. Using a spiralizer or a vegetable peeler, create zucchini noodles from the zucchinis.

2. Heat olive oil in a skillet over medium heat. Add the minced garlic and sauté for about 1 minute until fragrant.

3. Add the zucchini noodles to the skillet and sauté for 2•3 minutes, or until they are just tender.

4. Pour the marinara sauce over the zucchini noodles and toss to combine. Heat through.
5. Season with salt and pepper to taste.

6. Serve the zucchini noodles with marinara sauce hot, garnished with grated Parmesan cheese and fresh basil leaves.

This zucchini noodles with marinara sauce dish is low in fat and carbohydrates, making it a light and flavorful option for those following a no gallbladder diet. Enjoy this healthy and satisfying meal!

12. Cottage cheese with sliced peaches

Ingredient:

- 1/2 cup cottage cheese
- 1 ripe peach, sliced
- Optional: a drizzle of honey or a sprinkle of cinnamon

Instructions:

1. Spoon the cottage cheese into a bowl.

2. Top the cottage cheese with the sliced peaches.

3. Drizzle a little honey or sprinkle cinnamon over the top, if desired, for added sweetness and flavor.

4. Enjoy this cottage cheese with sliced peaches as a light and satisfying snack or breakfast option.

Cottage cheese is a good source of protein and calcium, while peaches provide vitamins and fiber, making this combination a healthy and gallbladder•friendly choice. Enjoy this creamy and fruity treat!

13. Poached eggs on whole grain toast

Ingredient:

• 2 eggs
• 2 slices of whole grain bread, toasted
• Salt and pepper to taste
• Optional toppings: avocado slices, tomato slices, or fresh herbs

Instructions:

1. Fill a saucepan with water and bring it to a gentle simmer.

2. Crack each egg into a small bowl or ramekin.

3. Carefully slide each egg into the simmering water.

4. Poach the eggs for about 3•4 minutes, or until the whites are set but the yolks are still runny.

5. Using a slotted spoon, remove the poached eggs from the water and drain on a paper towel.

6. Place the toasted whole grain bread on a plate.

7. Gently place a poached egg on each slice of toast.

8. Season with salt and pepper to taste.

9. Add any optional toppings you desire, such as avocado slices, tomato slices, or fresh herbs.

10. Serve the poached eggs on whole grain toast hot as a nutritious and satisfying breakfast or meal option.

This dish is high in protein, fiber, and essential nutrients, making it a healthy and gallbladder•friendly choice. Enjoy this simple and delicious meal!

14. Baked chicken thighs with roasted Brussels sprouts

Ingredient:

• 4 chicken thighs, bone•in and skin•on
• 1 pound Brussels sprouts, trimmed and halved
• 2 tablespoons olive oil
• 2 cloves garlic, minced
• 1 teaspoon dried thyme
• Salt and pepper to taste
• Lemon wedges for serving

Instructions:

1. Preheat your oven to 400°F (200°C).

2. In a bowl, combine the olive oil, minced garlic, dried thyme, salt, and pepper.

3. Place the chicken thighs in a baking dish and brush them with the olive oil mixture.

4. Arrange the Brussels sprouts around the chicken thighs in the baking dish. Drizzle any remaining olive oil mixture over the Brussels sprouts.

5. Bake in the preheated oven for about 30•35 minutes, or until the chicken is cooked through and the Brussels sprouts are tender and caramelized.

6. Serve the baked chicken thighs with roasted Brussels sprouts hot, with lemon wedges on the side for extra flavor.

This dish is rich in protein, fiber, and vitamins, making it a healthy and gallbladder•friendly option. Enjoy this delicious and wholesome meal!

15. Tuna salad on mixed greens

Ingredient:

- 1 can of tuna, drained
- 2 cups mixed salad greens
- 1/4 cup cherry tomatoes, halved
- 1/4 cup cucumber, sliced
- 1/4 cup red onion, thinly sliced
- 1 tablespoon olive oil
- 1 tablespoon lemon juice
- Salt and pepper to taste
- Optional toppings: avocado slices, boiled egg slices, or olives

Instructions:

1. In a bowl, combine the drained tuna with olive oil, lemon juice, salt, and pepper.

2. Place the mixed salad greens on a plate.

3. Top the greens with the tuna mixture.

4. Add cherry tomatoes, cucumber slices, and red onion on top of the tuna.

5. Add any optional toppings you desire, such as avocado slices, boiled egg slices, or olives.

6. Drizzle a little extra olive oil and lemon juice over the salad, if desired.

7. Serve the tuna salad on mixed greens as a light and refreshing meal option.

This tuna salad on mixed greens is high in protein, vitamins, and minerals, making it a healthy and gallbladder•friendly choice. Enjoy this simple and flavorful salad!

16. Mashed sweet potatoes with grilled chicken breast

Ingredient:

• 2 medium sweet potatoes, peeled and cubed
• 2 boneless, skinless chicken breasts
• 2 tablespoons olive oil
• Salt and pepper to taste
• Optional seasonings for chicken: paprika, garlic powder, onion powder
• Fresh parsley for garnish

Instructions:

1. In a pot, boil the sweet potato cubes until they are tender, about 15•20 minutes. Drain and mash the sweet potatoes until smooth. Season with salt and pepper to taste.

2. Preheat your grill or grill pan to medium•high heat.

3. Season the chicken breasts with salt, pepper, and any optional seasonings you prefer.

4. Brush the chicken breasts with olive oil.

5. Grill the chicken breasts for about 6•7 minutes per side, or until they are cooked through and reach an internal temperature of 165°F (74°C).

6. Serve the grilled chicken breasts alongside the mashed sweet potatoes.

7. Garnish with fresh parsley before serving.

This meal is rich in protein, fiber, and vitamins, making it a healthy and gallbladder•friendly option. Enjoy this flavorful and satisfying dish!

17. Ratatouille (vegetable stew)

Ingredient:

- 1 eggplant, diced
- 2 zucchinis, diced
- 1 yellow bell pepper, diced
- 1 red bell pepper, diced
- 1 onion, diced
- 2 cloves garlic, minced
- 2 tomatoes, diced
- 2 tablespoons olive oil
- 1 teaspoon dried thyme
- 1 teaspoon dried oregano
- Salt and pepper to taste
- Fresh basil for garnish

Instructions:

1. In a large pot or Dutch oven, heat olive oil over medium heat.

2. Add the diced onion and garlic, and sauté until softened and fragrant.

3. Add the diced eggplant, zucchinis, bell peppers, and tomatoes to the pot.

4. Season with dried thyme, dried oregano, salt, and pepper. Stir to combine.

5. Cover the pot and let the vegetables simmer over low heat for about 20•25 minutes, or until they are tender.

6. Adjust seasoning with salt and pepper if needed.

7. Serve the ratatouille hot, garnished with fresh basil.

Ratatouille is a flavorful and nutritious dish that is high in fiber and vitamins, making it a healthy and gallbladder•friendly option. Enjoy this hearty vegetable stew!

18. Smoothies with low•fat yogurt and mixed fruits

Ingredient:

• 1 cup low•fat yogurt
• 1 cup mixed fruits (such as berries, banana, mango, or pineapple)
• 1/2 cup liquid (water, almond milk, or coconut water)
• Optional add•ins: chia seeds, flaxseeds, or honey

Instructions:

1. In a blender, combine the low•fat yogurt, mixed fruits, and your choice of liquid.

2. Add any optional add•ins you desire, such as chia seeds, flaxseeds, or honey.

3. Blend until smooth and creamy.

4. Taste the smoothie and adjust sweetness if needed by adding more honey or fruits.

5. Pour the smoothie into a glass and enjoy it immediately as a healthy and satisfying snack or breakfast option.

This smoothie made with low•fat yogurt and mixed fruits is rich in protein, vitamins, and antioxidants, making it a nutritious and gallbladder•friendly choice. Enjoy this delicious and energizing drink!

19. Turkey chili with kidney beans

Ingredient:

• 1 pound ground turkey
• 1 can (15 oz) kidney beans, drained and rinsed
• 1 can (14.5 oz) diced tomatoes
• 1 onion, chopped
• 2 cloves garlic, minced
• 1 bell pepper, diced
• 1 tablespoon chili powder
• 1 teaspoon cumin
• Salt and pepper to taste
• Optional toppings: shredded cheese, chopped green onions, or Greek yogurt

Instructions:

1. In a large pot, cook the ground turkey over medium heat until browned.

2. Add the chopped onion, minced garlic, and diced bell pepper to the pot. Cook until the vegetables are softened.

3. Stir in the chili powder and cumin, and cook for another minute to toast the spices.

4. Add the diced tomatoes and kidney beans to the pot. Season with salt and pepper.

5. Bring the chili to a simmer, then reduce heat and let it simmer for about 20•30 minutes to allow the flavors to meld together.

6. Adjust seasoning with salt and pepper if needed.

7. Serve the turkey chili hot, garnished with shredded cheese, chopped green onions, or a dollop of Greek yogurt.

This turkey chili with kidney beans is high in protein and fiber, making it a healthy and gallbladder•friendly option. Enjoy this comforting and satisfying chili!

20. Steamed fish with ginger and soy sauce

Ingredient:

• 2 fish fillets (such as tilapia, cod, or salmon)
• 2 tablespoons soy sauce
• 1 tablespoon fresh ginger, grated
• 1 clove garlic, minced
• 1 green onion, chopped
• 1 tablespoon sesame oil
• Salt and pepper to taste
• Optional garnish: fresh cilantro leaves

Instructions:
1. Season the fish fillets with salt and pepper.

2. In a small bowl, mix together the soy sauce, grated ginger, minced garlic, chopped green onion, and sesame oil.

3. Place the fish fillets on a heatproof dish suitable for steaming.

4. Pour the soy sauce mixture over the fish fillets, making sure they are well coated.

5. Prepare a steamer and steam the fish fillets for about 8•10 minutes, or until the fish is cooked through and flakes easily with a fork.

6. Carefully remove the dish from the steamer.

7. Garnish the steamed fish with fresh cilantro leaves before serving.

This steamed fish with ginger and soy sauce dish is low in fat and high in protein, making it a healthy and gallbladder•friendly option. Enjoy this delicate and aromatic fish dish!

2I. Quinoa stuffed bell peppers

Ingredient:

• 4 bell peppers, tops removed and seeds removed
• 1 cup quinoa, cooked
• 1 can (15 oz) black beans, drained and rinsed
• 1 cup corn kernels
• 1 can (14.5 oz) diced tomatoes
• 1 teaspoon cumin
• 1 teaspoon chili powder
• Salt and pepper to taste
• Optional toppings: shredded cheese, avocado slices, or fresh cilantro

Instructions:

1. Preheat your oven to 375°F (190°C).

2. In a large bowl, mix together the cooked quinoa, black beans, corn kernels, diced tomatoes, cumin, chili powder, salt, and pepper.

3. Stuff each bell pepper with the quinoa mixture and place them in a baking dish.

4. Cover the baking dish with foil and bake in the preheated oven for about 25•30 minutes, or until the bell peppers are tender.

5. Remove the foil and sprinkle shredded cheese on top of each stuffed bell pepper, if desired.

6. Return the baking dish to the oven and bake for an additional 5 minutes, or until the cheese is melted.

7. Serve the quinoa stuffed bell peppers hot, garnished with avocado slices and fresh cilantro.

This dish is high in fiber, protein, and essential nutrients, making it a healthy and gallbladder•friendly option. Enjoy these delicious and colorful quinoa stuffed bell peppers!

22. Egg drop soup with vegetables

Ingredient:

• 4 cups chicken or vegetable broth
• 2 eggs, beaten
• 1 cup mixed vegetables (such as carrots, peas, corn)
• 2 green onions, chopped
• 1 tablespoon soy sauce
• 1 teaspoon sesame oil
• Salt and pepper to taste

Instructions:

1. In a pot, bring the chicken or vegetable broth to a simmer over medium heat.

2. Add the mixed vegetables to the broth and cook until they are tender.

3. In a small bowl, whisk together the beaten eggs.

4. Slowly pour the beaten eggs into the simmering broth while stirring gently with a fork to create egg ribbons.

5. Stir in the chopped green onions, soy sauce, sesame oil, salt, and pepper.

6. Taste the soup and adjust seasoning if needed.

7. Serve the egg drop soup with vegetables hot as a light and nourishing meal option.

This egg drop soup with vegetables is low in fat and high in protein and vitamins, making it a healthy and gallbladder•friendly choice. Enjoy this simple and satisfying soup!

23. Grilled chicken and vegetable kebabs

Ingredient:

• 2 boneless, skinless chicken breasts, cut into cubes
• Assorted vegetables (such as bell peppers, zucchini, cherry tomatoes, mushrooms)
• 2 tablespoons olive oil
• 2 cloves garlic, minced
• 1 teaspoon dried herbs (such as oregano, thyme, or rosemary)
• Salt and pepper to taste
• Wooden skewers, soaked in water

Instructions:

1. In a bowl, combine the olive oil, minced garlic, dried herbs, salt, and pepper.

2. Add the chicken cubes to the bowl and toss to coat evenly. Marinate for about 15•20 minutes.

3. Preheat your grill to medium•high heat.

4. Thread the marinated chicken cubes and assorted vegetables onto the soaked wooden skewers, alternating between chicken and vegetables.

5. Grill the kebabs for about 10•12 minutes, turning occasionally, until the chicken is cooked through and the vegetables are tender and slightly charred.

6. Serve the grilled chicken and vegetable kebabs hot as a flavorful and satisfying meal option.

These grilled chicken and vegetable kebabs are high in protein, fiber, and nutrients, making them a healthy and gallbladder•friendly choice. Enjoy these colorful and tasty kebabs!

24. Baked tofu with stir•fried broccoli

Ingredient:

• 1 block of firm tofu, pressed and cut into cubes
• 2 tablespoons of soy sauce
• 1 tablespoon of olive oil
• 1 teaspoon of garlic powder
• 1 teaspoon of onion powder
• 1 teaspoon of paprika
• Salt and pepper to taste
• 2 cups of broccoli florets
• 1 tablespoon of sesame oil
• 2 cloves of garlic, minced
• 1 teaspoon of grated ginger
• 2 tablespoons of low•sodium soy sauce
• 1 tablespoon of rice vinegar
• 1 teaspoon of cornstarch mixed with 2 tablespoons of water

Instructions:

1. Preheat the oven to 400°F (200°C).

2. In a bowl, mix together the soy sauce, olive oil, garlic powder, onion powder, paprika, salt, and pepper. Add the tofu cubes and toss to coat.

3. Place the tofu cubes on a baking sheet lined with parchment paper. Bake for 25•30 minutes, flipping halfway through, until the tofu is golden and crispy.

4. In a large skillet, heat the sesame oil over medium heat. Add the garlic and ginger and sauté for 1•2 minutes until fragrant.

5. Add the broccoli florets to the skillet and stir•fry for 5•7 minutes until tender•crisp.

6. In a small bowl, mix together the low•sodium soy sauce, rice vinegar, and cornstarch slurry. Pour the sauce over the broccoli and toss to coat. Cook for another 2•3 minutes until the sauce thickens. Serve the baked tofu with the stir•fried broccoli on the side. Enjoy your meal!

This recipe is low in fat and easy to digest, making it suitable for a no gallbladder diet. Enjoy your meal!

25. Spinach salad with grilled salmon

Ingredient:

• 1 lb salmon fillet
• 2 tablespoons olive oil
• 1 teaspoon garlic powder
• 1 teaspoon paprika
• Salt and pepper to taste
• 6 cups fresh spinach leaves
• 1 cup cherry tomatoes, halved
• 1/2 red onion, thinly sliced
• 1/4 cup feta cheese, crumbled
• 1/4 cup toasted pine nuts
• Lemon wedges for serving

For the dressing:
• 3 tablespoons olive oil
• 2 tablespoons balsamic vinegar
• 1 teaspoon Dijon mustard
• 1 teaspoon honey
• Salt and pepper to taste

Instructions:

1. Preheat the grill to medium•high heat.

2. In a small bowl, mix together the olive oil, garlic powder, paprika, salt, and pepper. Brush the mixture over the salmon fillet.

3. Grill the salmon for 4•5 minutes per side, or until cooked through. Remove from the grill and let it rest for a few minutes before flaking it into large pieces.

4. In a large salad bowl, combine the spinach leaves, cherry tomatoes, red onion, feta cheese, and pine nuts.

5. In a small jar, combine the olive oil, balsamic vinegar, Dijon mustard, honey, salt, and pepper. Shake well to emulsify the dressing.

6. Drizzle the dressing over the salad and toss to combine. Divide the salad onto plates and top with the grilled salmon pieces.

8. Serve with lemon wedges on the side for squeezing over the salmon. Enjoy your delicious and nutritious Spinach Salad with Grilled Salmon!

26. Bean and vegetable burritos with low•fat cheese

Ingredient:

• 1 can of low•sodium black beans, drained and rinsed
• 1 red bell pepper, diced
• 1 yellow bell pepper, diced
• 1 small zucchini, diced
• 1 small onion, diced
• 2 cloves of garlic, minced
• 1 teaspoon chili powder
• 1 teaspoon cumin
• Salt and pepper to taste
• 4 whole wheat tortillas
• 1 cup low•fat shredded cheese
• Salsa, avocado, and Greek yogurt for serving (optional)

Instructions:

1. In a large skillet, heat some olive oil over medium heat. Add the diced onion and garlic and sauté until softened.

2. Add the diced bell peppers and zucchini to the skillet and cook until they start to soften.

3. Add the drained black beans, chili powder, cumin, salt, and pepper to the skillet. Stir well to combine and cook for a few more minutes until the vegetables are tender.

4. Preheat the oven to 350°F (175°C).

5. Place a scoop of the bean and vegetable mixture onto each whole wheat tortilla. Top with a sprinkle of low•fat shredded cheese.

6. Roll up the tortillas, tucking in the sides as you go, to form burritos.

7. Place the burritos on a baking sheet lined with parchment paper. Bake in the preheated oven for about 10•15 minutes, or until the cheese is melted and the burritos are heated through.

8. Serve the bean and vegetable burritos with salsa, avocado slices, and a dollop of Greek yogurt if desired. Enjoy your flavorful and nutritious Bean and Vegetable Burritos with Low•Fat Cheese!

This recipe is low in fat and high in fiber, making it a suitable option for a no gallbladder diet. It's a delicious and satisfying meal that is easy to digest and packed with healthy ingredients.

27. Baked pork tenderloin with applesauce

Ingredient:

- 1 lb pork tenderloin
- 1 tablespoon olive oil
- 1 teaspoon garlic powder
- 1 teaspoon dried thyme
- Salt and pepper to taste
- 1 cup unsweetened applesauce
- 1 tablespoon honey
- 1 teaspoon Dijon mustard
- 1/2 teaspoon cinnamon

Instructions:

1. Preheat the oven to 375°F (190°C).

2. In a small bowl, mix together the olive oil, garlic powder, dried thyme, salt, and pepper. Rub the mixture over the pork tenderloin.

3. Place the seasoned pork tenderloin in a baking dish and bake in the preheated oven for about 25·30 minutes, or until the internal temperature reaches 145°F (63°C).

4. While the pork is baking, prepare the applesauce glaze. In a small saucepan, combine the unsweetened applesauce, honey, Dijon mustard, and cinnamon. Heat over low heat, stirring occasionally, until warmed through.

5. Once the pork tenderloin is cooked, remove it from the oven and let it rest for a few minutes before slicing.

6. Serve the sliced pork tenderloin with the warm applesauce glaze drizzled on top.

7. Enjoy your delicious and tender Baked Pork Tenderloin with Applesauce!

This recipe is low in fat and easy to digest, making it suitable for a no gallbladder diet. The combination of savory pork with sweet and tangy applesauce creates a flavorful and comforting dish that is gentle on the digestive system.

28. Shrimp and avocado salad

Ingredient:

- 1 lb large shrimp, peeled and deveined
- 1 tablespoon olive oil
- 1 teaspoon paprika
- Salt and pepper to taste
- 4 cups mixed salad greens
- 1 avocado, diced
- 1/2 cup cherry tomatoes, halved
- 1/4 red onion, thinly sliced
- 1/4 cup fresh cilantro, chopped
- 1/4 cup feta cheese, crumbled
- Lemon wedges for serving

For the dressing:
- 3 tablespoons olive oil
- 2 tablespoons lemon juice
- 1 teaspoon Dijon mustard
- 1 teaspoon honey
- Salt and pepper to taste

Instructions:

1. In a bowl, toss the shrimp with olive oil, paprika, salt, and pepper until well coated.

2. Heat a skillet over medium•high heat and cook the shrimp for 2•3 minutes per side, or until pink and cooked through. Remove from heat and set aside.

3. In a large salad bowl, combine the mixed salad greens, diced avocado, cherry tomatoes, red onion, cilantro, and feta cheese.

4. In a small jar, combine the olive oil, lemon juice, Dijon mustard, honey, salt, and pepper. Shake well to emulsify the dressing.

5. Drizzle the dressing over the salad and toss to combine. Divide the salad onto plates and top with the cooked shrimp.

7. Serve with lemon wedges on the side for squeezing over the salad. Enjoy your fresh and flavorful Shrimp and Avocado Salad!

This recipe is light, nutritious, and easy to digest, making it suitable for a no gallbladder diet. The combination of protein•rich shrimp, creamy avocado, and fresh vegetables makes for a satisfying and delicious meal option.

29. Whole wheat pasta with marinara sauce

Ingredient:

- 8 oz whole wheat pasta
- 2 tablespoons olive oil
- 2 cloves garlic, minced
- 1/2 onion, diced
- 1 can (14 oz) crushed tomatoes
- 1 teaspoon dried oregano
- 1 teaspoon dried basil
- Salt and pepper to taste
- Fresh basil leaves for garnish
- Grated Parmesan cheese (optional)

Instructions:

1. Cook the whole wheat pasta according to the package instructions until al dente. Drain and set aside.

2. In a large skillet, heat the olive oil over medium heat. Add the minced garlic and diced onion and sauté until softened and fragrant.

3. Add the crushed tomatoes, dried oregano, dried basil, salt, and pepper to the skillet. Stir well to combine.

4. Simmer the marinara sauce for about 15·20 minutes, stirring occasionally, to allow the flavors to meld together.

5. Add the cooked whole wheat pasta to the skillet with the marinara sauce. Toss to coat the pasta evenly with the sauce.

6. Serve the whole wheat pasta with marinara sauce in bowls, garnished with fresh basil leaves and grated Parmesan cheese if desired. Enjoy your simple and delicious Whole Wheat Pasta with Marinara Sauce!

This recipe is low in fat and easy to digest, making it suitable for a no gallbladder diet. Whole wheat pasta provides fiber and nutrients, while the marinara sauce is light and flavorful, making it a satisfying and comforting meal option.

30. Vegetable curry with chicken or tofu

Ingredient:

• 1 lb boneless, skinless chicken breast (or firm tofu for a vegetarian option), cut into cubes
• 2 tablespoons olive oil
• 1 onion, diced
• 2 cloves garlic, minced
• 1 tablespoon curry powder
• 1 teaspoon ground cumin
• 1 teaspoon ground coriander
• 1 teaspoon turmeric
• 1 can (14 oz) coconut milk
• 1 cup vegetable broth
• 2 cups mixed vegetables (such as bell peppers, carrots, peas, and broccoli)
• Salt and pepper to taste
• Fresh cilantro for garnish
• Cooked rice or naan bread for serving

Instructions:

1. In a large skillet or pot, heat the olive oil over medium heat. Add the diced onion and minced garlic and sauté until softened and fragrant.

2. Add the chicken cubes (or tofu cubes) to the skillet and cook until browned on all sides.

3. Stir in the curry powder, cumin, coriander, and turmeric, and cook for another minute to toast the spices.

4. Pour in the coconut milk and vegetable broth, stirring to combine. Bring the mixture to a simmer.

5. Add the mixed vegetables to the skillet and simmer for about 15•20 minutes, or until the chicken is cooked through (or tofu is heated) and the vegetables are tender. Season the curry with salt and pepper to taste.

5. Serve the vegetable curry with chicken or tofu over cooked rice or with naan bread. Garnish with fresh cilantro before serving. Enjoy your flavorful and comforting Vegetable Curry with Chicken or Tofu!

This recipe is rich in flavor and nutrients, making it a satisfying and nourishing meal option suitable for a no gallbladder diet. The combination of protein, vegetables, and aromatic spices makes this dish a delicious and wholesome choice.

31. Baked tilapia with lemon and herbs

Ingredient:

• 4 tilapia fillets
• 2 tablespoons olive oil
• 2 cloves garlic, minced
• 1 teaspoon dried thyme
• 1 teaspoon dried oregano
• Salt and pepper to taste
• 1 lemon, sliced
• Fresh parsley for garnish

Instructions:

1. Preheat the oven to 400°F (200°C).

2. In a small bowl, mix together the olive oil, minced garlic, dried thyme, dried oregano, salt, and pepper.

3. Place the tilapia fillets on a baking sheet lined with parchment paper.

4. Brush the olive oil and herb mixture over the tilapia fillets, coating them evenly.

5. Place lemon slices on top of each tilapia fillet.

6. Bake in the preheated oven for about 12•15 minutes, or until the tilapia is cooked through and flakes easily with a fork.

7. Remove from the oven and garnish with fresh parsley.

8. Serve the Baked Tilapia with Lemon and Herbs with a side of steamed vegetables or a salad. Enjoy your light and flavorful meal!

This recipe is low in fat and easy to digest, making it suitable for a no gallbladder diet. Tilapia is a mild and lean fish that pairs well with the bright flavors of lemon and herbs, creating a delicious and healthy dish that is gentle on the digestive system.

32. Hummus with raw vegetables

Ingredient:

• 1 can (15 oz) chickpeas, drained and rinsed
• 2 tablespoons tahini
• 2 cloves garlic, minced
• 2 tablespoons lemon juice
• 2 tablespoons olive oil
• 1/2 teaspoon cumin
• Salt and pepper to taste
• Raw vegetables for dipping (such as carrot sticks, cucumber slices, bell pepper strips, and cherry tomatoes)

Instructions:

1. In a food processor, combine the chickpeas, tahini, minced garlic, lemon juice, olive oil, cumin, salt, and pepper.

2. Blend the ingredients until smooth and creamy, adding a little water if needed to reach your desired consistency.

3. Taste the hummus and adjust the seasoning if necessary.

4. Transfer the hummus to a serving bowl and drizzle with a little extra olive oil.

5. Arrange the raw vegetables around the hummus for dipping.

6. Serve the Hummus with Raw Vegetables as a healthy and flavorful snack or appetizer.
7. Enjoy the creamy hummus with the crisp and fresh raw vegetables!

This recipe is low in fat and high in fiber, making it suitable for a no gallbladder diet. Hummus is a nutritious and delicious dip that pairs well with a variety of raw vegetables, providing a satisfying and healthy snack option that is easy on the digestive system.

33. Turkey lettuce wraps with shredded carrots and cucumber

Ingredient:

- 1 lb ground turkey
- 1 tablespoon olive oil
- 2 cloves garlic, minced
- 1 teaspoon ginger, grated
- 2 tablespoons low•sodium soy sauce
- 1 tablespoon hoisin sauce
- 1 teaspoon sesame oil
- 1 head of iceberg or butter lettuce, leaves separated
- 1/2 cup shredded carrots
- 1/2 cup shredded cucumber
- Fresh cilantro leaves for garnish
- Sriracha sauce (optional)

Instructions:

1. In a large skillet, heat the olive oil over medium heat. Add the minced garlic and grated ginger and sauté until fragrant.

2. Add the ground turkey to the skillet and cook until browned and cooked through.

3. Stir in the low•sodium soy sauce, hoisin sauce, and sesame oil. Cook for another 2•3 minutes to allow the flavors to meld.

4. Arrange the lettuce leaves on a serving platter.

5. Spoon the cooked turkey mixture onto each lettuce leaf.

6. Top the turkey with shredded carrots and cucumber.

7. Garnish with fresh cilantro leaves and drizzle with sriracha sauce if desired.

8. Serve the Turkey Lettuce Wraps with Shredded Carrots and Cucumber as a light and flavorful meal. Enjoy the delicious and nutritious lettuce wraps!

This recipe is low in fat and high in protein, making it suitable for a no gallbladder diet. The fresh and crunchy vegetables add texture and flavor to the savory turkey filling, creating a satisfying and healthy dish that is easy to digest.

34. Cauliflower rice stir•fry with chicken and snap peas

Ingredient:

• 1 lb boneless, skinless chicken breast, cut into strips
• 1 head of cauliflower, riced
• 2 tablespoons olive oil
• 2 cloves garlic, minced
• 1 tablespoon ginger, grated
• 1 cup snap peas
• 1 carrot, julienned
• 1 red bell pepper, sliced
• 2 tablespoons low•sodium soy sauce
• 1 tablespoon oyster sauce
• Salt and pepper to taste
• Green onions for garnish

Instructions:

1. In a large skillet or wok, heat 1 tablespoon of olive oil over medium•high heat. Add the chicken strips and cook until browned and cooked through. Remove the chicken from the skillet and set aside.

2. In the same skillet, add the remaining olive oil. Add the minced garlic and grated ginger and sauté until fragrant.

3. Add the snap peas, julienned carrot, and sliced red bell pepper to the skillet. Stir•fry for a few minutes until the vegetables are tender•crisp.

4. Push the vegetables to one side of the skillet and add the riced cauliflower to the other side. Cook the cauliflower for a few minutes until heated through.

5. Return the cooked chicken to the skillet and mix everything together.

6. In a small bowl, mix together the low•sodium soy sauce and oyster sauce. Pour the sauce over the stir•fry and toss to coat.

7. Season with salt and pepper to taste. Garnish with chopped green onions before serving. Enjoy your flavorful and healthy Cauliflower Rice Stir•Fry with Chicken and Snap Peas!

This recipe is low in fat and carbohydrates, making it suitable for a no gallbladder diet. Cauliflower rice is a great alternative to traditional rice and pairs well with the tender chicken and crunchy vegetables in this delicious stir•fry.

35. Bean soup with carrots and celery

Ingredient:

• 1 cup dried beans (such as navy beans, cannellini beans, or chickpeas), soaked overnight and drained
• 1 tablespoon olive oil
• 1 onion, diced
• 2 carrots, diced
• 2 stalks celery, diced
• 2 cloves garlic, minced
• 6 cups vegetable broth
• 1 teaspoon dried thyme
• 1 teaspoon dried rosemary
• Salt and pepper to taste
• Fresh parsley for garnish

Instructions:

1. In a large pot, heat the olive oil over medium heat. Add the diced onion, carrots, celery, and garlic. Sauté until the vegetables are softened.

2. Add the soaked and drained beans to the pot.

3. Pour in the vegetable broth and add the dried thyme and rosemary.

4. Bring the soup to a boil, then reduce the heat to low and simmer for about 1•2 hours, or until the beans are tender.

5. Season the soup with salt and pepper to taste.

6. Using an immersion blender, partially blend the soup to thicken it while still leaving some whole beans and vegetables for texture.

7. Serve the Bean Soup with Carrots and Celery hot, garnished with fresh parsley. Enjoy your hearty and nutritious bean soup!

This recipe is high in fiber and plant•based protein, making it a healthy and satisfying option suitable for a no gallbladder diet. The combination of beans, carrots, and celery provides a variety of nutrients and flavors in this comforting and nourishing soup.

36. Grilled portobello mushrooms with quinoa and spinach

Ingredient:

• 4 large portobello mushrooms
• 1/4 cup balsamic vinegar
• 2 tablespoons olive oil
• 2 cloves garlic, minced
• Salt and pepper to taste
• 1 cup quinoa, rinsed
• 2 cups vegetable broth
• 2 cups fresh spinach
• 1/4 cup pine nuts, toasted
• Fresh parsley for garnish

Instructions:

1. In a shallow dish, whisk together the balsamic vinegar, olive oil, minced garlic, salt, and pepper. Place the portobello mushrooms in the marinade, turning to coat. Let them marinate for about 30 minutes.

2. Preheat the grill to medium heat. Grill the marinated portobello mushrooms for about 4•5 minutes per side, or until tender.

3. In a saucepan, bring the vegetable broth to a boil. Add the rinsed quinoa, reduce the heat to low, cover, and simmer for about 15•20 minutes, or until the quinoa is cooked and the liquid is absorbed.

4. In a large skillet, wilt the fresh spinach over medium heat.

5. Fluff the cooked quinoa with a fork and stir in the wilted spinach.

6. Toast the pine nuts in a dry skillet over medium heat until golden brown.

7. Serve the grilled portobello mushrooms on a bed of quinoa and spinach mixture.

8. Sprinkle with toasted pine nuts and garnish with fresh parsley. Enjoy your flavorful and nutritious Grilled Portobello Mushrooms with Quinoa and Spinach!

This recipe is low in fat and high in fiber and nutrients, making it a healthy and satisfying option suitable for a no gallbladder diet. The combination of grilled portobello mushrooms, quinoa, spinach, and pine nuts creates a delicious and wholesome meal that is gentle on the digestive system.

37. Baked sweet potato with cottage cheese and chives

Ingredient:

• 2 medium sweet potatoes
• 1 cup low•fat cottage cheese
• 2 tablespoons chopped chives
• Salt and pepper to taste
• Olive oil (optional)

Instructions:

1. Preheat the oven to 400°F (200°C).

2. Wash the sweet potatoes and pierce them several times with a fork.

3. Place the sweet potatoes on a baking sheet and bake for about 45•60 minutes, or until they are tender when pierced with a fork.

4. Remove the sweet potatoes from the oven and let them cool slightly.

5. Cut each sweet potato in half lengthwise and fluff the flesh with a fork.

6. Top each sweet potato half with a dollop of low•fat cottage cheese.

7. Sprinkle chopped chives over the cottage cheese.

8. Season with salt and pepper to taste.

9. Drizzle with a little olive oil if desired.

10. Serve the Baked Sweet Potatoes with Cottage Cheese and Chives as a nutritious and satisfying meal or side dish. Enjoy your delicious and wholesome baked sweet potatoes!

This recipe is low in fat and high in fiber and nutrients, making it a healthy and easy•to•digest option suitable for a no gallbladder diet. The combination of sweet potatoes, cottage cheese, and chives creates a flavorful and comforting dish that is gentle on the digestive system.

38. Broiled lamb chops with steamed green beans

Ingredient:

• 4 lamb chops
• 2 tablespoons olive oil
• 2 cloves garlic, minced
• 1 teaspoon dried rosemary
• Salt and pepper to taste
• 1 lb green beans, trimmed
• Lemon wedges for serving

Instructions:

1. Preheat the broiler in your oven.

2. In a small bowl, mix together the olive oil, minced garlic, dried rosemary, salt, and pepper.

3. Rub the mixture over the lamb chops, coating them evenly.

4. Place the seasoned lamb chops on a broiler pan or baking sheet.

5. Broil the lamb chops for about 4•5 minutes on each side, or until they reach your desired level of doneness.

6. While the lamb chops are broiling, steam the green beans until they are tender•crisp.

7. Season the green beans with a little salt and pepper.

8. Serve the broiled lamb chops with the steamed green beans on the side.

9. Garnish with lemon wedges for squeezing over the lamb chops.

10. Enjoy your delicious and savory Broiled Lamb Chops with Steamed Green Beans!

This recipe is rich in protein and nutrients, making it a satisfying and flavorful meal option. The combination of tender lamb chops with fresh green beans creates a balanced and nutritious dish that is suitable for a variety of dietary preferences, including a no gallbladder diet.

39. Chicken and vegetable skewers with brown rice

Ingredient:

• 1 lb boneless, skinless chicken breast, cut into cubes
• 1 red bell pepper, cut into chunks
• 1 yellow bell pepper, cut into chunks
• 1 zucchini, sliced
• 1 red onion, cut into chunks
• 2 tablespoons olive oil
• 2 cloves garlic, minced
• 1 teaspoon dried oregano
• Salt and pepper to taste
• Wooden skewers, soaked in water

For the brown rice:
• 1 cup brown rice
• 2 cups water
• Salt to taste

Instructions:

1. In a bowl, combine the olive oil, minced garlic, dried oregano, salt, and pepper. Add the chicken cubes and vegetables to the bowl and toss to coat.

2. Thread the marinated chicken and vegetables onto the soaked wooden skewers, alternating between the chicken and vegetables.

3. Preheat a grill or grill pan over medium•high heat.

4. Grill the skewers for about 10•12 minutes, turning occasionally, until the chicken is cooked through and the vegetables are tender.

5. While the skewers are grilling, rinse the brown rice under cold water. In a saucepan, combine the brown rice, water, and salt. Bring to a boil, then reduce the heat to low, cover, and simmer for about 40•45 minutes, or until the rice is tender and the water is absorbed.

6. Serve the Chicken and Vegetable Skewers with the cooked brown rice on the side. Enjoy your flavorful and nutritious meal!

This recipe is a balanced and healthy option that combines lean protein from the chicken with a variety of colorful vegetables and whole grains from the brown rice. It's a satisfying and delicious dish that is suitable for a no gallbladder diet.

40. Spinach and feta stuffed chicken breast

Ingredient:

• 4 boneless, skinless chicken breasts
• 2 cups fresh spinach, chopped
• 1/2 cup crumbled feta cheese
• 2 cloves garlic, minced
• 1 tablespoon olive oil
• 1 teaspoon dried oregano
• Salt and pepper to taste
• Toothpicks or kitchen twine

Instructions:

1. Preheat the oven to 375°F (190°C).

2. In a skillet, heat the olive oil over medium heat. Add the minced garlic and chopped spinach. Cook until the spinach is wilted.

3. Remove the skillet from heat and stir in the crumbled feta cheese. Allow the mixture to cool slightly.

4. Butterfly each chicken breast by slicing horizontally through the middle, but not all the way through, to create a pocket.

5. Season the inside of each chicken breast with salt, pepper, and dried oregano.

6. Stuff each chicken breast with the spinach and feta mixture, then secure the opening with toothpicks or kitchen twine. Season the outside of the chicken breasts with a little more salt, pepper, and oregano.

8. Place the stuffed chicken breasts in a baking dish and bake in the preheated oven for about 25•30 minutes, or until the chicken is cooked through. Remove the toothpicks or twine before serving.

10. Serve the Spinach and Feta Stuffed Chicken Breast with a side of vegetables or salad. Enjoy your delicious and flavorful stuffed chicken breasts!

This recipe combines tender chicken breasts with a savory spinach and feta filling, creating a tasty and satisfying dish that is suitable for a no gallbladder diet. It's a nutritious and easy•to•make meal option that is sure to impress your taste buds.

41. Greek salad with grilled chicken

Ingredient:

- 1 lb boneless, skinless chicken breasts
- 2 tablespoons olive oil
- 2 cloves garlic, minced
- 1 teaspoon dried oregano
- Salt and pepper to taste
- 4 cups mixed salad greens
- 1 cucumber, diced
- 1 cup cherry tomatoes, halved

- 1/2 red onion, thinly sliced
- 1/2 cup Kalamata olives, pitted
- 1/2 cup crumbled feta cheese
- Lemon wedges for serving

For the dressing:
- 1/4 cup olive oil
- 2 tablespoons red wine vinegar
- 1 teaspoon dried oregano
- Salt and pepper to taste

Instructions:

1. In a bowl, mix together the olive oil, minced garlic, dried oregano, salt, and pepper. Add the chicken breasts and toss to coat. Let them marinate for about 30 minutes.

2. Preheat a grill or grill pan over medium•high heat. Grill the chicken breasts for about 6•7 minutes per side, or until cooked through. Remove from the grill and let them rest for a few minutes before slicing.

3. In a large salad bowl, combine the mixed salad greens, diced cucumber, cherry tomatoes, red onion, Kalamata olives, and crumbled feta cheese.

4. In a small jar, combine the olive oil, red wine vinegar, dried oregano, salt, and pepper. Shake well to emulsify the dressing.

5. Drizzle the dressing over the salad and toss to combine.

6. Divide the salad onto plates and top with the sliced grilled chicken.

7. Serve the Greek Salad with Grilled Chicken with lemon wedges on the side for squeezing over the salad. Enjoy your fresh and flavorful Greek salad with tender grilled chicken!

This recipe is rich in protein, fiber, and healthy fats, making it a nutritious and satisfying meal option suitable for a no gallbladder diet. The combination of fresh vegetables, tangy feta cheese, and grilled chicken creates a delicious and balanced dish that is gentle on the digestive system.

42. Tofu and vegetable stir•fry with brown rice

Ingredient:

- 1 block of firm tofu, pressed and cubed
- 2 tablespoons soy sauce
- 1 tablespoon sesame oil
- 1 tablespoon cornstarch
- 2 tablespoons vegetable oil
- 2 cloves garlic, minced
- 1 tablespoon ginger, grated

- 1 red bell pepper, sliced
- 1 cup broccoli florets
- 1 carrot, sliced
- 1/2 cup snap peas
- 1/4 cup low•sodium vegetable broth
- 2 tablespoons hoisin sauce
- Cooked brown rice for serving

Instructions:

1. In a bowl, mix the cubed tofu with soy sauce, sesame oil, and cornstarch until well coated.

2. Heat vegetable oil in a large skillet or wok over medium•high heat. Add the tofu and cook until golden brown on all sides. Remove from the skillet and set aside.

3. In the same skillet, add a little more oil if needed. Add the minced garlic and grated ginger, and sauté for about 1 minute until fragrant.

4. Add the sliced red bell pepper, broccoli florets, carrot, and snap peas to the skillet. Stir•fry for a few minutes until the vegetables are tender•crisp.

5. In a small bowl, mix the vegetable broth and hoisin sauce. Pour the sauce over the vegetables in the skillet.

6. Add the cooked tofu back to the skillet and toss everything together to coat in the sauce.

7. Serve the tofu and vegetable stir•fry over cooked brown rice. Enjoy your delicious and nutritious Tofu and Vegetable Stir•Fry with Brown Rice!

This recipe is high in plant•based protein, fiber, and nutrients, making it a healthy and satisfying meal option suitable for a no gallbladder diet. The combination of tofu, colorful vegetables, and flavorful sauce over brown rice creates a balanced and delicious dish that is gentle on the digestive system.

43. Baked acorn squash with lean ground turkey and cranberries

Ingredient:

• 2 acorn squash, halved and seeds removed
• 1 lb lean ground turkey
• 1 tablespoon olive oil
• 1 small onion, diced
• 2 cloves garlic, minced
• 1 teaspoon dried sage
• 1/2 teaspoon dried thyme
• Salt and pepper to taste
• 1/2 cup dried cranberries
• 1/4 cup chopped pecans (optional)
• Fresh parsley for garnish

Instructions:

1. Preheat the oven to 400°F (200°C).

2. Place the acorn squash halves cut side down on a baking sheet. Bake for about 30•40 minutes, or until the squash is tender when pierced with a fork.

3. In a skillet, heat the olive oil over medium heat. Add the diced onion and minced garlic, and sauté until softened.

4. Add the lean ground turkey to the skillet and cook until browned and cooked through.

5. Stir in the dried sage, dried thyme, salt, and pepper. Add the dried cranberries and chopped pecans to the skillet and mix well. Once the acorn squash is baked, remove it from the oven and flip the halves over.

6. Fill each acorn squash half with the ground turkey mixture. Return the stuffed acorn squash to the oven and bake for an additional 10•15 minutes. Garnish with fresh parsley before serving.

7. Enjoy your flavorful and festive Baked Acorn Squash with Lean Ground Turkey and Cranberries!

This recipe combines the natural sweetness of acorn squash with savory lean ground turkey, tart cranberries, and crunchy pecans for a delicious and nutritious meal. It's a comforting and satisfying dish that is suitable for a no gallbladder diet.

44. Low•fat yogurt parfait with granola and fresh fruit

Ingredient:

• 1 cup low•fat or fat•free yogurt
• 1/2 cup granola (choose a low•fat or low•sugar option)
• 1/2 cup fresh mixed berries (such as strawberries, blueberries, raspberries)
• 1 tablespoon honey (optional)
• Fresh mint leaves for garnish

Instructions:

1. In a glass or bowl, layer the low•fat or fat•free yogurt with granola and fresh mixed berries.

2. Drizzle a little honey over the top if desired for added sweetness.

3. Repeat the layers until you reach the top of the glass or bowl.

4. Garnish with fresh mint leaves for a pop of color and freshness.

5. Serve the Low•Fat Yogurt Parfait with Granola and Fresh Fruit as a nutritious and delicious breakfast, snack, or dessert option.

6. Enjoy your light and satisfying parfait!

This recipe is low in fat and easy to digest, making it suitable for a no gallbladder diet. The combination of creamy yogurt, crunchy granola, and sweet fresh fruit creates a balanced and flavorful parfait that is rich in nutrients and fiber. It's a refreshing and satisfying option that can be enjoyed at any time of the day.

45. Baked eggplant Parmesan with minimal cheese

Ingredient:

• 1 large eggplant, sliced into rounds
• 1 cup whole wheat breadcrumbs
• 1/2 cup grated Parmesan cheese
• 1 teaspoon dried oregano
• 1 teaspoon dried basil
• Salt and pepper to taste
• 2 eggs, beaten
• Olive oil cooking spray
• Marinara sauce (store•bought or homemade)
• Fresh basil leaves for garnish

Instructions:

1. Preheat the oven to 400°F (200°C).

2. In a shallow dish, mix together the whole wheat breadcrumbs, grated Parmesan cheese, dried oregano, dried basil, salt, and pepper.

3. Dip each eggplant slice into the beaten eggs, then coat with the breadcrumb mixture, pressing gently to adhere.

4. Place the coated eggplant slices on a baking sheet lined with parchment paper.

5. Lightly spray the tops of the eggplant slices with olive oil cooking spray.

6. Bake in the preheated oven for about 20•25 minutes, or until the eggplant is tender and the coating is crispy.

7. Remove the baked eggplant slices from the oven and top each slice with a spoonful of marinara sauce. Sprinkle a little more Parmesan cheese on top of each slice.

8. Return the baking sheet to the oven and bake for an additional 5•10 minutes, or until the cheese is melted and bubbly. Garnish with fresh basil leaves before serving. Enjoy your light and flavorful Baked Eggplant Parmesan with Minimal Cheese!

This recipe is low in fat and uses whole wheat breadcrumbs and minimal cheese, making it suitable for a no gallbladder diet. The baked eggplant slices are crispy on the outside and tender on the inside, topped with marinara sauce and a sprinkle of Parmesan cheese for a delicious and satisfying dish.

46. Chicken and barley soup with carrots and onions

Ingredient:

• 1 lb boneless, skinless chicken breast, diced
• 1 cup pearl barley
• 2 carrots, diced
• 1 onion, diced
• 2 cloves garlic, minced
• 6 cups low•sodium chicken broth
• 1 teaspoon dried thyme
• Salt and pepper to taste
• Fresh parsley for garnish

Instructions:

1. In a large pot, heat a little olive oil over medium heat. Add the diced chicken breast and cook until browned.

2. Add the diced onion and minced garlic to the pot and sauté until fragrant.

3. Stir in the pearl barley and diced carrots.

4. Pour in the low•sodium chicken broth and add the dried thyme, salt, and pepper.

5. Bring the soup to a boil, then reduce the heat to low, cover, and simmer for about 45•50 minutes, or until the barley is tender and the chicken is cooked through.

6. Adjust the seasoning with salt and pepper to taste.

7. Serve the Chicken and Barley Soup with Carrots and Onions hot, garnished with fresh parsley. Enjoy your hearty and nutritious soup!

This recipe is low in fat and high in fiber and protein, making it a healthy and satisfying option suitable for a no gallbladder diet. The combination of tender chicken, hearty barley, and flavorful vegetables creates a comforting and nourishing soup that is gentle on the digestive system.

47. Grilled turkey burgers with lettuce wraps

Ingredient:

• 1 lb ground turkey
• 1/4 cup breadcrumbs
• 1 egg
• 1/2 teaspoon garlic powder
• 1/2 teaspoon onion powder
• 1/2 teaspoon dried oregano
• Salt and pepper to taste
• Lettuce leaves for wrapping
• Optional toppings: sliced tomatoes, red onion, avocado, mustard, ketchup

Instructions:

1. In a bowl, combine the ground turkey, breadcrumbs, egg, garlic powder, onion powder, dried oregano, salt, and pepper. Mix until well combined.

2. Divide the turkey mixture into equal portions and shape into burger patties.

3. Preheat the grill to medium•high heat.

4. Grill the turkey burgers for about 5•6 minutes per side, or until they are cooked through and reach an internal temperature of 165°F (74°C).

5. Remove the turkey burgers from the grill and let them rest for a few minutes.

6. To assemble the lettuce wraps, place a turkey burger on a lettuce leaf and top with your choice of toppings.

7. Wrap the lettuce around the burger like a taco and secure with a toothpick if needed.

8. Serve the Grilled Turkey Burgers with Lettuce Wraps as a light and flavorful meal.

9. Enjoy your delicious and healthy turkey burger lettuce wraps!

This recipe is low in fat and carbohydrates, making it a nutritious and satisfying option suitable for a no gallbladder diet. The lettuce wraps provide a refreshing and crunchy alternative to traditional burger buns, while the grilled turkey burgers offer a lean and flavorful protein option.

48. Steamed mussels with garlic and herbs

Ingredient:

• 2 lbs fresh mussels, cleaned and debearded
• 2 tablespoons olive oil
• 4 cloves garlic, minced
• 1/2 cup white wine
• 1/4 cup chopped fresh parsley
• 1 tablespoon chopped fresh thyme
• Salt and pepper to taste
• Lemon wedges for serving
• Crusty bread for dipping

Instructions:

1. In a large pot or Dutch oven, heat the olive oil over medium heat. Add the minced garlic and sauté for about 1 minute until fragrant.

2. Pour in the white wine and bring it to a simmer.

3. Add the cleaned mussels to the pot and sprinkle with chopped parsley, thyme, salt, and pepper.

4. Cover the pot with a lid and steam the mussels for about 5•7 minutes, or until they have opened.

5. Discard any mussels that have not opened.

6. Serve the steamed mussels in a large bowl, drizzled with the cooking liquid and herbs.

7. Serve with lemon wedges on the side for squeezing over the mussels.

8. Enjoy your flavorful and aromatic Steamed Mussels with Garlic and Herbs with some crusty bread for dipping!

This recipe is low in fat and high in protein, making it a healthy and delicious option suitable for a no gallbladder diet. The combination of fresh mussels, garlic, herbs, and white wine creates a flavorful and satisfying dish that is gentle on the digestive system.

49. Quinoa and black bean salad with lime dressing

Ingredient:

- 1 cup cooked quinoa, cooled
- 1 (15 oz) can black beans, rinsed and drained
- 1 cup diced cucumber
- 1/2 cup diced red onion
- 1/2 cup diced bell pepper
- 2 tablespoons chopped cilantro
- Juice of 1 lime
- 2 tablespoons olive oil
- 1 teaspoon honey
- Salt and pepper to taste

Instructions:

1. In a large bowl, combine the cooked quinoa, black beans, cucumber, red onion, bell pepper, and cilantro.

2. In a small bowl, whisk together the lime juice, olive oil, and honey. Season with salt and pepper.

3. Pour the dressing over the quinoa and bean mixture and toss gently to coat.

4. Refrigerate for at least 30 minutes to allow the flavors to meld.

This salad is a great option for a no gallbladder diet as it is low in fat and high in fiber, protein, and nutrients. The lime dressing provides a bright, tangy flavor without any heavy or creamy ingredients that could be difficult to digest. Enjoy!

50. Egg white and vegetable frittata with tomatoes and spinach

Ingredient:

- 8 egg whites
- 1/4 cup unsweetened almond milk
- 1/4 tsp salt
- 1/4 tsp black pepper
- 1 tbsp olive oil
- 1/2 cup diced onion
- 2 cloves garlic, minced
- 1 cup chopped fresh spinach
- 1 cup diced tomatoes
- 1/4 cup crumbled feta cheese (optional)

Instructions:

1. Preheat oven to 375°F.

2. In a medium bowl, whisk together the egg whites, almond milk, salt, and pepper.

3. Heat the olive oil in a 9•inch oven•safe nonstick skillet over medium heat. Add the onion and garlic and sauté for 2•3 minutes until translucent.

4. Add the spinach and tomatoes to the skillet and cook for 1•2 minutes until the spinach is wilted.

5. Pour the egg white mixture over the vegetables in the skillet. Use a spatula to gently lift the edges to allow the uncooked egg to flow underneath.

6. Transfer the skillet to the preheated oven and bake for 12•15 minutes, until the frittata is set.

7. Remove from oven and let cool for 5 minutes. Slice and serve, optionally topped with crumbled feta cheese.

This frittata is high in protein from the egg whites, and the vegetables provide fiber, vitamins, and minerals without any heavy or high•fat ingredients that could be difficult to digest for someone without a gallbladder.

51. Baked stuffed peppers with quinoa and ground turkey

Ingredient:

• 4 bell peppers, halved lengthwise and seeds/membranes removed
• 1 lb ground turkey
• 1 cup cooked quinoa
• 1 small onion, diced
• 2 cloves garlic, minced
• 1 (14.5 oz) can diced tomatoes
• 1 tsp dried oregano
• 1/2 tsp dried basil
• Salt and pepper to taste
• 1/4 cup shredded mozzarella cheese (optional)

Instructions:

1. Preheat oven to 375°F.

2. In a large skillet over medium heat, cook the ground turkey, onion, and garlic until the turkey is browned and the vegetables are softened, about 5•7 minutes. Drain any excess fat.

3. Stir in the cooked quinoa, diced tomatoes, oregano, basil, salt, and pepper. Simmer for 5 minutes.

4. Arrange the bell pepper halves in a baking dish. Spoon the turkey•quinoa mixture evenly into the pepper halves.

5. Cover the baking dish with foil and bake for 25•30 minutes, until the peppers are tender.

6. Remove the foil and sprinkle the tops of the stuffed peppers with the shredded mozzarella cheese, if using.

7. Return to the oven and bake for an additional 5•10 minutes, until the cheese is melted and bubbly. Serve hot.

This dish is a great option for a no gallbladder diet as it is low in fat and high in fiber, protein, and nutrients from the quinoa, ground turkey, and vegetables. The baked peppers provide a flavorful and satisfying vessel for the filling.

52. Grilled halibut with mango salsa

Ingredient:

For the Mango Salsa:
• 1 ripe mango, diced
• 1/2 red onion, finely chopped
• 1 jalapeño, seeded and finely chopped
• 1/4 cup chopped fresh cilantro
• Juice of 1 lime
• Salt and pepper to taste

For the Halibut:
• 4 (6 oz) halibut fillets
• 1 tbsp olive oil
• Salt and pepper to taste

Instructions:

1. Make the mango salsa: In a medium bowl, combine the diced mango, red onion, jalapeño, cilantro, and lime juice. Season with salt and pepper to taste. Cover and refrigerate until ready to serve.

2. Preheat grill or grill pan to medium•high heat.

3. Pat the halibut fillets dry and brush both sides with olive oil. Season generously with salt and pepper.

4. Grill the halibut for 4•5 minutes per side, or until it flakes easily with a fork and is opaque throughout.

5. Serve the grilled halibut immediately, topped with the chilled mango salsa.

This dish is perfect for a no gallbladder diet. Halibut is a lean, mild white fish that is easy to digest. The mango salsa provides a fresh, flavorful topping without any heavy sauces or creams. The meal is high in protein, low in fat, and full of vitamins and antioxidants from the mango, onion, and cilantro.

53. Stir•fried tofu with bok choy and soy sauce

Ingredient:

• 1 block (14 oz) firm or extra•firm tofu, cubed
• 2 tbsp low•sodium soy sauce
• 1 tbsp rice vinegar
• 1 tsp sesame oil
• 1 tbsp vegetable oil
• 3 cloves garlic, minced
• 1 inch piece fresh ginger, peeled and minced
• 4 cups chopped bok choy
• 2 green onions, sliced
• Salt and pepper to taste

Instructions:

1. In a small bowl, whisk together the soy sauce, rice vinegar, and sesame oil. Set aside.

2. Heat the vegetable oil in a large skillet or wok over medium•high heat. Add the tofu cubes and cook, stirring occasionally, until lightly browned on all sides, about 5•7 minutes. Transfer the tofu to a plate.

3. Add the garlic and ginger to the skillet and cook for 1 minute, until fragrant.

4. Add the bok choy and soy sauce mixture to the skillet. Cook, stirring frequently, until the bok choy is tender•crisp, about 3•4 minutes.

5. Return the cooked tofu to the skillet and toss everything together until heated through, about 2 more minutes.

6. Remove from heat and stir in the sliced green onions. Season with salt and pepper to taste.

7. Serve immediately over steamed brown rice or quinoa.

This stir•fry is a great option for a no gallbladder diet. The tofu provides lean protein, while the bok choy and other vegetables are high in fiber and nutrients. The soy sauce and sesame oil add flavor without any heavy or creamy ingredients that could be difficult to digest.

54. Greek yogurt with sliced almonds and honey

Ingredient:

• 1 cup plain Greek yogurt
• 2 tablespoons sliced almonds
• 1 tablespoon honey

Instructions:
1. Scoop the Greek yogurt into a bowl.

2. Sprinkle the sliced almonds over the top of the yogurt.

3. Drizzle the honey over the almonds and yogurt.

4. Serve immediately.

This snack or light meal is perfect for a no gallbladder diet for a few reasons:

1. Greek yogurt is low in fat and high in protein, which can be easier to digest for those without a gallbladder.

2. Almonds are a healthy source of fats, fiber, and nutrients. The sliced almonds provide a nice crunch without being too heavy.

3. Honey is a natural sweetener that is gentle on the digestive system, unlike refined sugars.

The combination of the creamy yogurt, crunchy almonds, and sweet honey creates a satisfying and nutritious snack that is easy to digest. This can be enjoyed on its own or paired with some fresh fruit for added fiber and vitamins.

55. Spaghetti squash
with marinara sauce and lean ground beef

Ingredient:

• 1 medium spaghetti squash, halved lengthwise and seeds removed
• 1 lb lean ground beef (93% lean or higher)
• 1 onion, diced
• 3 cloves garlic, minced
• 1 (28 oz) can crushed tomatoes
• 2 tbsp tomato paste
• 1 tsp dried oregano
• 1 tsp dried basil
• Salt and pepper to taste
• Grated Parmesan cheese (optional)

Instructions:

1. Preheat oven to 400°F. Place the spaghetti squash halves cut•side down on a baking sheet. Roast for 40•50 minutes, until tender when pierced with a fork.

2. Meanwhile, in a large skillet over medium•high heat, cook the ground beef, onion, and garlic until the beef is browned and the vegetables are softened, about 5•7 minutes. Drain any excess fat.

3. Stir in the crushed tomatoes, tomato paste, oregano, and basil. Season with salt and pepper to taste. Simmer the sauce for 10•15 minutes.

4. Once the spaghetti squash is cooked, use a fork to scrape the flesh into strands, creating "noodles."

5. Divide the spaghetti squash noodles between plates or bowls. Top with the marinara meat sauce.

6. Optionally, sprinkle with grated Parmesan cheese before serving.

This dish is a great option for a no gallbladder diet. The spaghetti squash provides fiber and nutrients without the heaviness of traditional pasta. The lean ground beef adds protein, while the tomato•based sauce is gentle on the digestive system. Overall, it's a nutritious and easy•to•digest meal.

56. Roasted chicken breast with butternut squash

Ingredient:

• 4 boneless, skinless chicken breasts
• 1 medium butternut squash, peeled, seeded, and cubed
• 2 tbsp olive oil
• 1 tsp dried thyme
• 1 tsp garlic powder
• Salt and pepper to taste

Instructions:

1. Preheat oven to 400°F.

2. In a large bowl, toss the cubed butternut squash with 1 tbsp of the olive oil, 1/2 tsp of the thyme, and a pinch of salt and pepper.

3. Spread the seasoned butternut squash cubes out on a large baking sheet. Roast for 20•25 minutes, stirring halfway, until the squash is tender and lightly browned.

4. Meanwhile, in the same bowl, toss the chicken breasts with the remaining 1 tbsp olive oil, 1/2 tsp thyme, garlic powder, and salt and pepper to taste.

5. Remove the baking sheet with the roasted squash from the oven. Push the squash to the sides of the sheet to make room for the chicken breasts.

6. Place the seasoned chicken breasts on the baking sheet with the squash.

7. Return the baking sheet to the oven and roast for an additional 20•25 minutes, until the chicken is cooked through and the juices run clear.

8. Serve the roasted chicken breast immediately, with the roasted butternut squash on the side.

This dish is perfect for a no gallbladder diet. The chicken breast is a lean protein that is easy to digest, while the butternut squash provides fiber, vitamins, and complex carbohydrates. The simple seasoning keeps the flavors light and fresh. This makes for a nutritious and satisfying meal.

57. Turkey sausage and vegetable stir•fry

Ingredient:

• 1 lb turkey sausage, sliced into 1/2•inch pieces
• 2 tbsp olive oil
• 1 red bell pepper, sliced
• 1 cup broccoli florets
• 1 cup sliced mushrooms
• 1 cup snow peas
• 3 cloves garlic, minced
• 1 tbsp low•sodium soy sauce
• 1 tsp sesame oil
• Salt and pepper to taste
• Cooked brown rice or quinoa, for serving

Instructions:

1. Heat the olive oil in a large skillet or wok over medium•high heat. Add the turkey sausage and cook, stirring occasionally, until lightly browned, about 5 minutes.

2. Add the bell pepper, broccoli, mushrooms, and snow peas to the skillet. Stir•fry for 3•4 minutes, until the vegetables are tender•crisp.

3. Add the minced garlic and cook for 1 minute, until fragrant.

4. Drizzle the soy sauce and sesame oil over the stir•fry and toss to coat everything evenly. Season with salt and pepper to taste.

5. Serve the turkey sausage and vegetable stir•fry immediately over cooked brown rice or quinoa.

This stir•fry is a great option for a no gallbladder diet. The turkey sausage provides lean protein, while the variety of vegetables add fiber, vitamins, and minerals. The soy sauce and sesame oil add flavor without any heavy or creamy ingredients that could be difficult to digest. Serving it over a whole grain like brown rice or quinoa makes it a complete and satisfying meal.

58. Baked trout with herb butter

Ingredient:

• 4 (6 oz) trout fillets
• 2 tbsp unsalted butter, softened
• 2 tbsp chopped fresh parsley
• 1 tbsp chopped fresh dill
• 1 tsp lemon zest
• 1/4 tsp salt
• 1/4 tsp black pepper

Instructions:

1. Preheat oven to 400°F. Line a baking sheet with parchment paper.

2. In a small bowl, mix together the softened butter, parsley, dill, lemon zest, salt, and pepper until well combined.

3. Place the trout fillets on the prepared baking sheet. Spread the herb butter evenly over the top of each fillet.

4. Bake for 12•15 minutes, until the trout is opaque and flakes easily with a fork.

5. Serve the baked trout immediately, with any extra herb butter spooned over the top.

This baked trout dish is an excellent option for a no gallbladder diet for a few reasons:

• Trout is a lean, mild•flavored fish that is easy to digest. It's high in protein and omega•3 fatty acids.

• The herb butter adds flavor without being heavy or creamy, which can be difficult for those without a gallbladder.

• Baking the fish keeps it light and simple, without the need for frying or sauces that may be harder to digest.

• The fresh herbs and lemon zest provide bright, fresh flavors that complement the trout nicely.

Serve this baked trout with a side of roasted vegetables or a simple salad for a complete and gallbladder•friendly meal.

59. Vegetable and lentil stew

Ingredient:

- 1 tbsp olive oil
- 1 onion, diced
- 3 cloves garlic, minced
- 2 carrots, peeled and diced
- 2 celery stalks, diced
- 1 cup green or brown lentils, rinsed
- 4 cups low•sodium vegetable broth
- 1 (14.5 oz) can diced tomatoes
- 2 cups chopped kale or spinach
- 1 tsp dried thyme
- 1 tsp dried oregano
- Salt and pepper to taste

Instructions:

1. In a large pot or Dutch oven, heat the olive oil over medium heat. Add the onion and sauté for 3•4 minutes until translucent.

2. Add the garlic, carrots, and celery. Cook for 5 more minutes, stirring occasionally.

3. Stir in the lentils, vegetable broth, diced tomatoes, kale/spinach, thyme, and oregano. Season with salt and pepper.

4. Bring the stew to a boil, then reduce heat and let simmer for 20•25 minutes, until the lentils are tender.

5. Taste and adjust seasoning as needed.

6. Serve the vegetable and lentil stew hot, garnished with extra chopped kale or parsley if desired.

This stew is an excellent option for a no gallbladder diet. It's packed with fiber•rich vegetables and protein•packed lentils, which are easy to digest. The tomatoes provide lycopene, while the greens offer vitamins and minerals. The simple seasoning avoids any heavy or creamy ingredients that could be difficult to digest. This makes for a nourishing, gallbladder•friendly meal.

60. Chicken Caesar salad with light dressing

Ingredient:

• 4 boneless, skinless chicken breasts
• 1 romaine lettuce heart, chopped
• 1 cup cherry tomatoes, halved
• 1/4 cup shredded Parmesan cheese
• 2 tbsp whole wheat croutons (optional)

For the Dressing:
• 1/4 cup plain Greek yogurt
• 2 tbsp lemon juice
• 1 tbsp Dijon mustard
• 1 garlic clove, minced
• 1 tsp Worcestershire sauce
• 2 tbsp olive oil
• Salt and pepper to taste

Instructions:

1. Preheat oven to 400°F. Season the chicken breasts with salt and pepper. Bake for 20•25 minutes until cooked through. Let cool, then slice or shred the chicken.

2. In a small bowl, whisk together the yogurt, lemon juice, Dijon, garlic, Worcestershire, and olive oil. Season with salt and pepper.

3. In a large salad bowl, combine the chopped romaine, tomatoes, Parmesan, and cooked chicken.

4. Drizzle the light Caesar dressing over the salad and toss gently to coat.

5. Top with whole wheat croutons if desired.

This chicken Caesar salad is a great option for a no gallbladder diet. The lean chicken breast provides protein, while the romaine lettuce, tomatoes, and Parmesan offer fiber, vitamins, and minerals. The light dressing, made with Greek yogurt instead of heavy mayo or cream, is easy to digest. This makes for a satisfying and nutritious meal.

61. Quinoa stuffed mushrooms with spinach and feta

Ingredient:

• 12 large mushrooms, stems removed and finely chopped
• 1 cup cooked quinoa
• 1 cup fresh spinach, chopped
• 1/4 cup crumbled feta cheese
• 2 tbsp olive oil
• 2 cloves garlic, minced
• 1/4 tsp dried oregano
• Salt and pepper to taste

Instructions:

1. Preheat oven to 375°F. Lightly grease a baking sheet.

2. In a medium skillet, heat the olive oil over medium heat. Add the chopped mushroom stems, garlic, and oregano. Sauté for 3•4 minutes until the mushrooms are softened.

3. Remove the skillet from heat and stir in the cooked quinoa, spinach, and feta cheese. Season with salt and pepper.

4. Stuff the mushroom caps evenly with the quinoa mixture, packing it in gently.

5. Arrange the stuffed mushrooms on the prepared baking sheet.

6. Bake for 15•18 minutes, until the mushrooms are tender and the filling is hot.

7. Serve the quinoa stuffed mushrooms warm.

This recipe is a great option for a no gallbladder diet for a few reasons:

• Mushrooms are low in fat and easy to digest.
• Quinoa is a high•protein, high•fiber grain that is gentle on the digestive system.
• Spinach provides fiber, vitamins, and minerals without any heavy sauces or creams.
• Feta cheese adds flavor without being too rich or heavy.

The simple preparation and baking method also makes this dish easy to digest. Enjoy these quinoa stuffed mushrooms as a healthy appetizer or light main course.

62. Ratatouille with chickpeas

Ingredient:

• 1 medium eggplant, diced
• 1 zucchini, diced
• 1 yellow squash, diced
• 1 red bell pepper, diced
• 1 onion, diced
• 3 cloves garlic, minced
• 1 (15 oz) can chickpeas, rinsed and drained
• 1 (14.5 oz) can diced tomatoes
• 2 tbsp olive oil
• 1 tsp dried thyme
• 1 tsp dried oregano
• Salt and pepper to taste
• Chopped fresh basil for garnish (optional)

Instructions:

1. In a large skillet or Dutch oven, heat the olive oil over medium heat. Add the diced eggplant, zucchini, squash, bell pepper, onion, and garlic. Sauté for 8•10 minutes, stirring occasionally, until the vegetables are tender.

2. Stir in the chickpeas, diced tomatoes, thyme, oregano, and a pinch of salt and pepper.

3. Reduce heat to medium•low and let the ratatouille simmer for 15•20 minutes, stirring occasionally, until the flavors have melded and the vegetables are very soft.

4. Taste and adjust seasoning as needed, adding more salt, pepper, or herbs to your preference.

5. Serve the ratatouille warm, garnished with chopped fresh basil if desired. Can be served over quinoa or brown rice.

This ratatouille with chickpeas is an excellent choice for a no gallbladder diet. The vegetables provide fiber, vitamins, and antioxidants, while the chickpeas add plant•based protein. The simple seasoning avoids any heavy or creamy sauces that could be difficult to digest. Overall, it's a nutritious, flavorful, and easy•to•digest vegetarian dish.

63. Egg white scramble with peppers and onions

Ingredient:

• 8 egg whites
• 1/4 cup unsweetened almond milk
• 1 tbsp olive oil
• 1/2 cup diced bell pepper (any color)
• 1/4 cup diced onion
• 1 clove garlic, minced
• Salt and pepper to taste
• 2 tbsp chopped fresh parsley (optional)

Instructions:

1. In a medium bowl, whisk together the egg whites and almond milk. Season with a pinch of salt and pepper.

2. Heat the olive oil in a nonstick skillet over medium heat. Add the diced bell pepper, onion, and garlic. Sauté for 3•4 minutes until the vegetables are softened.

3. Pour the egg white mixture into the skillet with the vegetables. Use a spatula to gently stir and scramble the eggs, cooking for 2•3 minutes until the eggs are cooked through but still moist.

4. Remove from heat and stir in the chopped parsley, if using.

5. Serve the egg white scramble immediately.

This egg white scramble is an excellent choice for a no gallbladder diet for a few reasons:

• Egg whites are a lean protein that is easy to digest.
• The vegetables (peppers and onions) provide fiber, vitamins, and minerals without any heavy or creamy ingredients.
• The simple seasoning with just salt, pepper, and optional parsley keeps the dish light and gentle on the digestive system.

This makes for a nutritious and satisfying breakfast or brunch option that is suitable for those following a no gallbladder diet. Pair it with a slice of whole grain toast or a side of roasted potatoes for a complete meal.

64. Baked cod with quinoa pilaf

Ingredient:

For the Quinoa Pilaf:
• 1 cup uncooked quinoa, rinsed
• 2 cups low•sodium vegetable or chicken broth
• 1 tbsp olive oil
• 1 onion, diced
• 2 cloves garlic, minced
• 1 cup diced bell pepper
• 1/4 cup chopped fresh parsley

For the Baked Cod:
• 4 (6 oz) cod fillets
• 1 tbsp olive oil
• 1 tsp paprika
• 1/2 tsp dried thyme
• Salt and pepper to taste

Instructions:
1. Preheat oven to 400°F. Lightly grease a baking sheet.

For the Quinoa Pilaf:
1. In a medium saucepan, combine the quinoa and broth. Bring to a boil, then reduce heat to low, cover, and simmer for 15•20 minutes until quinoa is tender.
2. In a skillet, heat the olive oil over medium heat. Add the onion, garlic, and bell pepper. Sauté for 5•7 minutes until softened.
3. Fluff the cooked quinoa with a fork and stir in the sautéed vegetables and chopped parsley. Season with salt and pepper.

For the Baked Cod:
1. Place the cod fillets on the prepared baking sheet. Drizzle with olive oil and sprinkle with paprika, thyme, salt, and pepper.
2. Bake for 12•15 minutes, until the cod is opaque and flakes easily with a fork.

To Serve:
1. Divide the quinoa pilaf evenly among 4 plates.
2. Top each portion of quinoa with a baked cod fillet.

This baked cod with quinoa pilaf is an excellent choice for a no gallbladder diet. The cod is a lean, mild fish that is easy to digest. The quinoa pilaf provides fiber, protein, and complex carbohydrates without any heavy sauces or creams. The simple seasoning keeps the dish light and flavorful.

65. Turkey and vegetable kebabs with tzatziki sauce

Ingredient:

For the Kebabs:
• 1 lb ground turkey
• 1 zucchini, cut into 1·inch pieces
• 1 red bell pepper, cut into 1·inch pieces
• 1 red onion, cut into 1·inch pieces
• 8 cherry tomatoes
• 2 tbsp olive oil
• 1 tsp dried oregano
• Salt and pepper to taste

For the Tzatziki Sauce:
• 1 cup plain Greek yogurt
• 1 cucumber, peeled, seeded, and grated
• 2 cloves garlic, minced
• 1 tbsp lemon juice
• 1 tbsp chopped fresh dill
• Salt and pepper to taste

Instructions:

1. Preheat grill or grill pan to medium·high heat.

For the Kebabs:
1. In a bowl, gently mix together the ground turkey, olive oil, oregano, salt, and pepper until well combined.
2. Thread the turkey mixture, zucchini, bell pepper, onion, and tomatoes onto skewers.
3. Grill the kebabs for 12·15 minutes, turning occasionally, until the turkey is cooked through and the vegetables are tender.

For the Tzatziki Sauce:
1. In a medium bowl, stir together the Greek yogurt, grated cucumber, garlic, lemon juice, dill, salt, and pepper.
2. Refrigerate the tzatziki sauce until ready to serve.

To Serve:
1. Arrange the grilled turkey and vegetable kebabs on a platter.
2. Serve the tzatziki sauce on the side for dipping.

This dish is perfect for a no gallbladder diet. The lean ground turkey and grilled vegetables are easy to digest, while the tzatziki sauce provides a refreshing, creamy topping without any heavy ingredients. The simple seasoning keeps the flavors light and fresh. Enjoy these turkey and vegetable kebabs as a healthy main course or appetizer.

66. Steamed shrimp with cocktail sauce

Ingredient:

For the Shrimp:
• 1 lb large shrimp, peeled and deveined
• 1 cup water
• 1 tbsp lemon juice

For the Cocktail Sauce:
• 1/2 cup ketchup
• 2 tbsp prepared horseradish
• 1 tbsp lemon juice
• 1 tsp Worcestershire sauce
• 1/4 tsp hot sauce (optional)
• Salt and pepper to taste

Instructions:

1. Fill a large pot with 1 cup of water and the 1 tbsp lemon juice. Bring to a boil over high heat.

2. Add the shrimp to the pot, cover, and steam for 3•5 minutes, until the shrimp are opaque and cooked through. Drain and transfer the shrimp to a serving platter.

For the Cocktail Sauce:
1. In a small bowl, whisk together the ketchup, horseradish, 1 tbsp lemon juice, Worcestershire sauce, and hot sauce (if using). Season with salt and pepper to taste.

2. Serve the steamed shrimp immediately with the cocktail sauce on the side for dipping.

This steamed shrimp with cocktail sauce is an excellent choice for a no gallbladder diet. The shrimp is a lean protein that is easy to digest, and the simple steaming method avoids any heavy or fried preparations.

The cocktail sauce is made with just a few simple ingredients • ketchup, horseradish, lemon juice, and Worcestershire • providing a flavorful dipping sauce without any creamy or fatty components that could be difficult to digest.

This makes for a light, healthy, and gallbladder•friendly appetizer or main course. Enjoy the shrimp with the zesty cocktail sauce for a delicious and digestible meal.

67. Chicken and vegetable curry with brown rice

Ingredient:

- 1 lb boneless, skinless chicken breasts, cubed
- 2 tbsp olive oil
- 1 onion, diced
- 3 cloves garlic, minced
- 1 tbsp grated fresh ginger
- 2 tsp curry powder
- 1 tsp ground cumin
- 1/2 tsp ground turmeric
- 1 cup low•sodium chicken broth
- 1 (14 oz) can diced tomatoes
- 1 cup diced carrots
- 1 cup diced cauliflower florets
- 1 cup frozen peas
- 1 cup cooked brown rice
- Salt and pepper to taste
- Chopped cilantro for garnish (optional)

Instructions:

1. In a large skillet or Dutch oven, heat the olive oil over medium heat. Add the chicken and cook for 3•4 minutes until lightly browned.

2. Add the onion, garlic, and ginger to the skillet. Cook for 2•3 minutes until fragrant.

3. Stir in the curry powder, cumin, and turmeric. Cook for 1 minute to toast the spices.

4. Pour in the chicken broth and diced tomatoes. Add the carrots, cauliflower, and peas.

5. Bring the curry to a simmer and cook for 15•20 minutes, until the vegetables are tender and the chicken is cooked through.

6. Taste and season with salt and pepper as needed. Serve the chicken and vegetable curry over cooked brown rice. Garnish with chopped cilantro if desired.

This curry dish is an excellent choice for a no gallbladder diet. The lean chicken breast provides protein, while the variety of vegetables add fiber, vitamins, and minerals. The spices add flavor without any heavy or creamy sauces that could be difficult to digest. Serving it over brown rice makes it a complete and satisfying meal.

68. Spinach and mushroom frittata

Ingredient:

• 8 eggs
• 1/4 cup unsweetened almond milk
• 1 tbsp olive oil
• 8 oz sliced mushrooms
• 1 cup fresh spinach, chopped
• 2 cloves garlic, minced
• 1/4 cup crumbled feta cheese (optional)
• Salt and pepper to taste

Instructions:

1. Preheat oven to 375°F. Grease a 9•inch oven•safe skillet or pie dish.

2. In a medium bowl, whisk together the eggs and almond milk. Season with a pinch of salt and pepper.

3. In the greased skillet, heat the olive oil over medium heat. Add the sliced mushrooms and sauté for 3•4 minutes until softened.

4. Add the chopped spinach and minced garlic to the skillet. Cook for 1•2 minutes until the spinach is wilted.

5. Pour the egg mixture over the vegetables in the skillet. Use a spatula to gently lift the edges, allowing the uncooked egg to flow underneath.

6. Sprinkle the crumbled feta cheese over the top, if using.

7. Transfer the skillet to the preheated oven and bake for 15•18 minutes, until the frittata is set in the center.

8. Remove from oven and let cool for 5 minutes before slicing and serving.

This spinach and mushroom frittata is an excellent choice for a no gallbladder diet. The eggs provide protein, while the spinach and mushrooms add fiber, vitamins, and minerals. The simple preparation with just a touch of olive oil and optional feta keeps the dish light and easy to digest. This makes for a nutritious and satisfying breakfast, brunch, or light meal.

69. Baked sweet potato with black beans and salsa

Ingredient:

• 4 medium sweet potatoes
• 1 (15 oz) can black beans, rinsed and drained
• 1 cup prepared salsa
• 2 tbsp chopped fresh cilantro (optional)
• Salt and pepper to taste

Instructions:

1. Preheat oven to 400°F. Pierce the sweet potatoes several times with a fork.

2. Place the sweet potatoes directly on the oven rack and bake for 45•60 minutes, until very soft when squeezed.

3. Remove the sweet potatoes from the oven and let cool for 5 minutes.

4. Slice each sweet potato in half lengthwise. Scoop out the flesh into a bowl, leaving a thin layer of sweet potato attached to the skin.

5. Mash the sweet potato flesh lightly with a fork. Stir in the rinsed and drained black beans.

6. Spoon the sweet potato and black bean mixture back into the potato skins.

7. Top each stuffed sweet potato half with 2•3 tablespoons of salsa.

8. Sprinkle the chopped cilantro over the top, if using.

9. Serve the baked sweet potatoes warm.

This dish is perfect for a no gallbladder diet. Sweet potatoes are easy to digest and high in fiber, while the black beans provide plant•based protein. The salsa adds flavor without any heavy sauces or creams. This makes for a nutritious, fiber•rich, and gallbladder•friendly meal.

70. Grilled pork tenderloin with apple slaw

Ingredient:

For the Pork Tenderloin:
• 1 lb pork tenderloin
• 1 tbsp olive oil
• 1 tsp garlic powder
• 1 tsp dried thyme
• Salt and pepper to taste

For the Apple Slaw:
• 2 cups shredded green cabbage
• 1 cup shredded red cabbage
• 1 Granny Smith apple, julienned
• 2 tbsp apple cider vinegar
• 1 tbsp olive oil
• 1 tsp Dijon mustard
• 1 tsp honey
• Salt and pepper to taste

Instructions:
For the Pork Tenderloin:
1. Preheat grill or grill pan to medium•high heat.
2. Rub the pork tenderloin all over with the olive oil, garlic powder, thyme, salt, and pepper.
3. Grill the pork for 12•15 minutes, turning occasionally, until it reaches an internal temperature of 145°F. Let the pork rest for 5 minutes before slicing.

For the Apple Slaw:
1. In a large bowl, combine the shredded green and red cabbage, and julienned apple.
2. In a small bowl, whisk together the apple cider vinegar, olive oil, Dijon mustard, and honey. Season with salt and pepper.
3. Pour the dressing over the cabbage and apple mixture and toss to coat.

To Serve:
1. Slice the grilled pork tenderloin.
2. Serve the pork slices alongside the apple slaw.

This grilled pork tenderloin with apple slaw is an excellent choice for a no gallbladder diet. Pork tenderloin is a lean protein that is easy to digest. The apple slaw provides fiber, vitamins, and a light, tangy flavor without any heavy creams or dressings. The simple seasoning and grilling method keeps the dish light and gallbladder•friendly.

71. Greek yogurt smoothie with berries and chia seeds

Ingredient:

• 1 cup plain Greek yogurt
• 1 cup mixed berries (such as blueberries, raspberries, strawberries)
• 1/2 cup unsweetened almond milk
• 1 tbsp chia seeds
• 1 tsp honey (optional)

Instructions:

1. In a blender, combine the Greek yogurt, mixed berries, almond milk, and chia seeds.

2. Blend on high speed until smooth and creamy, about 1 minute.

3. Taste and add 1 tsp of honey if you'd like it a bit sweeter.

4. Pour the smoothie into a glass and enjoy immediately.

This Greek yogurt smoothie is an excellent choice for a no gallbladder diet for several reasons:

• Greek yogurt is high in protein and low in fat, making it easy to digest.

• Berries are packed with fiber, vitamins, and antioxidants.

• Chia seeds provide additional fiber and healthy omega•3 fatty acids.

• Almond milk is a dairy•free, low•fat milk alternative.

• The honey is optional, but provides a touch of natural sweetness if desired.

The smooth, creamy texture of this smoothie makes it gentle on the digestive system, while the nutrient•dense ingredients provide sustained energy and nourishment. This makes for a great breakfast, snack, or light meal option for those following a no gallbladder diet.

72. Lemon garlic shrimp with steamed broccoli

Ingredient:

• 1 lb large shrimp, peeled and deveined
• 2 tbsp olive oil
• 3 cloves garlic, minced
• 1 tbsp lemon juice
• 1 tsp lemon zest
• 1/4 tsp red pepper flakes (optional)
• Salt and pepper to taste
• 4 cups broccoli florets
• 2 tbsp water

Instructions:

1. In a large skillet, heat the olive oil over medium heat. Add the minced garlic and sauté for 1 minute until fragrant.

2. Add the shrimp to the skillet and cook for 2•3 minutes per side, until the shrimp are opaque and cooked through.

3. Stir in the lemon juice, lemon zest, and red pepper flakes (if using). Season with salt and pepper.

4. Meanwhile, place the broccoli florets in a steamer basket set over a pot of simmering water. Steam for 5•7 minutes, until the broccoli is tender•crisp.

5. Serve the lemon garlic shrimp immediately, with the steamed broccoli on the side.

This dish is perfect for a no gallbladder diet. The shrimp provides lean protein that is easy to digest, while the broccoli offers fiber, vitamins, and minerals. The simple lemon and garlic flavors add taste without any heavy sauces or creams that could be difficult on the digestive system.

The steaming method for the broccoli also keeps it light and gentle on the stomach. This makes for a nutritious and gallbladder•friendly meal that is quick and easy to prepare.

73. Tofu lettuce wraps with hoisin sauce

Ingredient:

- 1 block (14 oz) extra•firm tofu, diced
- 1 tbsp sesame oil
- 2 cloves garlic, minced
- 1 tbsp grated fresh ginger
- 1/4 cup low•sodium soy sauce
- 2 tbsp hoisin sauce
- 1 cup shredded carrots
- 1 cup shredded cabbage
- 8•10 large lettuce leaves (such as romaine or bibb)
- Chopped green onions for garnish (optional)

Instructions:

1. In a large skillet or wok, heat the sesame oil over medium•high heat. Add the diced tofu and cook for 5•7 minutes, stirring occasionally, until lightly browned.

2. Add the minced garlic and grated ginger to the skillet. Cook for 1 minute until fragrant.

3. Stir in the soy sauce and hoisin sauce. Cook for 2•3 minutes, allowing the sauce to thicken slightly.

4. Remove the skillet from heat and stir in the shredded carrots and cabbage.

5. To serve, spoon the tofu and vegetable mixture into the lettuce leaves. Garnish with chopped green onions if desired.

This tofu lettuce wrap recipe is perfect for a no gallbladder diet. Tofu is a lean, plant•based protein that is easy to digest. The crunchy vegetables add fiber, while the hoisin sauce provides flavor without any heavy or creamy ingredients.

The lettuce leaves act as a light, low•calorie wrap, keeping the dish gentle on the digestive system. This makes for a nutritious, flavorful, and gallbladder•friendly meal or appetizer.

74. Quinoa tabbouleh with cucumber and tomatoes

Ingredient:

• 1 cup uncooked quinoa, rinsed
• 1 cup diced cucumber
• 1 cup diced tomatoes
• 1/2 cup chopped fresh parsley
• 1/4 cup chopped fresh mint
• 2 tbsp lemon juice
• 1 tbsp olive oil
• 1 clove garlic, minced
• 1/4 tsp ground cumin
• Salt and pepper to taste

Instructions:

1. Cook the quinoa according to package instructions. Fluff with a fork and let cool.

2. In a large bowl, combine the cooked quinoa, diced cucumber, diced tomatoes, chopped parsley, and chopped mint.

3. In a small bowl, whisk together the lemon juice, olive oil, minced garlic, and ground cumin. Season with salt and pepper.

4. Pour the dressing over the quinoa and vegetable mixture. Toss gently to coat everything evenly.

5. Refrigerate the quinoa tabbouleh for at least 30 minutes to allow the flavors to meld.

6. Serve chilled or at room temperature.

This quinoa tabbouleh is an excellent choice for a no gallbladder diet. Quinoa is a high•protein, high•fiber grain that is easy to digest. The fresh vegetables • cucumber, tomatoes, parsley, and mint • provide additional fiber, vitamins, and minerals without any heavy or creamy ingredients.

The simple lemon and olive oil dressing keeps the flavors light and refreshing. This makes for a nutritious, gallbladder•friendly salad or side dish that can be enjoyed on its own or paired with grilled lean protein.

75. Turkey chili with sweet potatoes

Ingredient:

• 1 lb ground turkey
• 1 onion, diced
• 3 cloves garlic, minced
• 2 medium sweet potatoes, peeled and diced
• 1 (15 oz) can diced tomatoes
• 1 (15 oz) can black beans, rinsed and drained
• 1 cup low•sodium chicken or vegetable broth
• 2 tbsp chili powder
• 1 tsp ground cumin
• 1 tsp dried oregano
• 1/4 tsp cayenne pepper (optional)
• Salt and pepper to taste
• Chopped fresh cilantro for garnish (optional)

Instructions:

1. In a large pot or Dutch oven, cook the ground turkey over medium•high heat, breaking it up with a wooden spoon, until browned, about 5•7 minutes. Drain any excess fat.

2. Add the diced onion and minced garlic to the pot. Cook for 2•3 minutes until fragrant.

3. Stir in the diced sweet potatoes, diced tomatoes, black beans, broth, chili powder, cumin, oregano, and cayenne (if using). Season with salt and pepper.

4. Bring the chili to a boil, then reduce heat and let simmer for 20•25 minutes, until the sweet potatoes are tender.

5. Taste and adjust seasonings as needed.

6. Serve the turkey and sweet potato chili hot, garnished with chopped fresh cilantro if desired.

This turkey chili is an excellent choice for a no gallbladder diet. The lean ground turkey provides protein, while the sweet potatoes offer complex carbohydrates, fiber, and vitamins. The simple spices add flavor without any heavy or creamy ingredients that could be difficult to digest.

The combination of protein, fiber, and complex carbs makes this chili a nutritious and satisfying meal that is gentle on the digestive system. Enjoy it on its own or serve over brown rice or quinoa.

76. Baked chicken thighs with cauliflower mash

Ingredient:

For the Chicken:
• 6 bone•in, skin•on chicken thighs
• 1 tbsp olive oil
• 1 tsp paprika
• 1 tsp garlic powder
• Salt and pepper to taste

For the Cauliflower Mash:
• 1 head of cauliflower, cut into florets
• 2 tbsp unsweetened almond milk
• 1 tbsp olive oil
• 2 cloves garlic, minced
• Salt and pepper to taste

Instructions:
For the Chicken:
1. Preheat oven to 400°F. Line a baking sheet with parchment paper.
2. Pat the chicken thighs dry and place them on the prepared baking sheet. Drizzle with olive oil and sprinkle with paprika, garlic powder, salt, and pepper.
3. Bake for 35•40 minutes, until the chicken is cooked through and the skin is crispy.

For the Cauliflower Mash:
1. In a large pot, bring a few inches of water to a boil. Add the cauliflower florets and steam for 8•10 minutes, until very tender.
2. Drain the cauliflower and transfer to a food processor. Add the almond milk, olive oil, and minced garlic. Pulse until smooth and creamy.
3. Season the cauliflower mash with salt and pepper to taste.

To Serve:
1. Serve the baked chicken thighs alongside the cauliflower mash.

This dish is perfect for a no gallbladder diet. The chicken thighs provide protein, while the cauliflower mash offers a low•carb, fiber•rich alternative to traditional mashed potatoes. The simple seasoning keeps the flavors light and easy to digest.

The baking method for the chicken and the smooth texture of the cauliflower mash make this a gentle, gallbladder•friendly meal. Enjoy this comforting and nutritious dish.

77. Stir•fried vegetables with tofu and teriyaki sauce

Ingredient:

• 1 block (14 oz) extra•firm tofu, cubed
• 2 tbsp low•sodium soy sauce
• 1 tbsp rice vinegar
• 1 tbsp honey
• 1 tsp sesame oil
• 2 tbsp olive oil
• 3 cloves garlic, minced
• 1 inch piece fresh ginger, peeled and grated
• 1 red bell pepper, sliced
• 1 cup broccoli florets
• 1 cup sliced mushrooms
• 2 cups baby spinach
• Salt and pepper to taste
• Chopped green onions for garnish (optional)

Instructions:

1. In a small bowl, whisk together the soy sauce, rice vinegar, honey, and sesame oil. Set the teriyaki•style sauce aside.

2. In a large skillet or wok, heat the olive oil over medium•high heat. Add the cubed tofu and cook for 3•4 minutes per side until lightly browned. Transfer the tofu to a plate.

3. In the same skillet, add the minced garlic and grated ginger. Cook for 1 minute until fragrant.

4. Add the sliced bell pepper, broccoli florets, and mushrooms to the skillet. Stir•fry for 3•4 minutes until the vegetables are tender•crisp.

5. Return the cooked tofu to the skillet and pour in the teriyaki•style sauce. Toss everything together and cook for 2•3 minutes until the sauce thickens slightly.

6. Remove from heat and stir in the baby spinach. Season with salt and pepper to taste. Serve the stir•fried vegetables and tofu immediately, garnished with chopped green onions if desired. Serve over steamed brown rice or quinoa.

This stir•fry is a great option for a no gallbladder diet. The tofu provides plant•based protein, while the vegetables offer fiber, vitamins, and minerals. The simple teriyaki•style sauce adds flavor without any heavy or creamy ingredients that could be difficult to digest.

78. Broiled salmon with quinoa and roasted vegetables

Ingredient:

• 4 salmon fillets (about 6 oz each)
• 1 cup quinoa, rinsed
• 2 cups low•sodium vegetable or chicken broth
• 1 lb mixed vegetables (such as broccoli, cauliflower, bell peppers, zucchini), chopped into 1•inch pieces
• 2 tbsp olive oil
• Salt and pepper to taste

Instructions:

1. Preheat oven to 400°F. Toss the chopped vegetables with 1 tbsp olive oil, salt, and pepper. Spread in a single layer on a baking sheet. Roast for 20•25 minutes, stirring halfway, until vegetables are tender and lightly browned.

2. While the vegetables are roasting, cook the quinoa. In a medium saucepan, combine the quinoa and broth. Bring to a boil, then reduce heat to low, cover and simmer for 15•20 minutes until quinoa is tender and liquid is absorbed. Fluff with a fork.

3. Brush the salmon fillets with the remaining 1 tbsp olive oil and season with salt and pepper.

4. Turn oven to broil. Place the salmon fillets on a foil•lined baking sheet. Broil for 8•10 minutes, flipping halfway, until salmon is opaque and flakes easily with a fork.

5. Serve the broiled salmon over the cooked quinoa, topped with the roasted vegetables.

This meal is high in protein, fiber, and healthy fats, while being low in fat and cholesterol • making it a great option for those following a no gallbladder diet.

79. Lentil and vegetable soup

Ingredient:

• 1 cup dried brown or green lentils, rinsed
• 6 cups low•sodium vegetable or chicken broth
• 1 tbsp olive oil
• 1 onion, diced
• 3 cloves garlic, minced
• 2 carrots, peeled and diced
• 2 celery stalks, diced
• 1 zucchini, diced
• 1 (14.5 oz) can diced tomatoes
• 2 tsp dried thyme
• 1 tsp dried oregano
• Salt and pepper to taste

Instructions:

1. In a large pot, bring the lentils and broth to a boil over high heat. Reduce heat to medium•low, cover and simmer for 15•20 minutes, until lentils are tender.

2. In a large skillet, heat the olive oil over medium heat. Add the onion and garlic and cook for 2•3 minutes until fragrant.

3. Add the carrots, celery and zucchini to the skillet. Cook for 5•7 minutes, stirring occasionally, until vegetables are starting to soften.

4. Add the cooked vegetables, diced tomatoes, thyme, oregano, salt and pepper to the pot with the cooked lentils. Stir to combine.

5. Bring the soup back to a simmer and cook for an additional 10•15 minutes, until vegetables are tender.

6. Taste and adjust seasoning as needed.

This lentil and vegetable soup is packed with fiber, protein, and nutrients, while being low in fat and cholesterol • making it a great option for those following a no gallbladder diet. The lentils provide a hearty, filling base, while the vegetables add flavor and texture.

80. Grilled turkey sausage
with sautéed peppers and onions

Ingredient:

• 4 turkey sausages (look for low•fat or lean varieties)
• 1 tbsp olive oil
• 1 red bell pepper, sliced
• 1 green bell pepper, sliced
• 1 onion, sliced
• 2 cloves garlic, minced
• Salt and pepper to taste

Instructions:

1. Preheat grill or grill pan to medium•high heat.

2. Grill the turkey sausages for 12•15 minutes, turning occasionally, until cooked through. Set aside.

3. In a large skillet, heat the olive oil over medium heat.

4. Add the sliced bell peppers and onion. Sauté for 5•7 minutes, stirring occasionally, until vegetables are starting to soften.

5. Add the minced garlic and continue cooking for 2•3 minutes more, until vegetables are tender.

6. Season the sautéed vegetables with salt and pepper to taste.

7. Serve the grilled turkey sausages topped with the sautéed peppers and onions.

This dish is a great option for those following a no gallbladder diet. Turkey sausage is a lean protein that is easy to digest, while the sautéed peppers and onions provide fiber, vitamins, and minerals without being too heavy or high in fat. The simple preparation makes this a quick and healthy meal.

81. Egg white and spinach omelette

Ingredient:

• 4 egg whites
• 1 cup fresh spinach, chopped
• 1 tbsp low•fat milk or unsweetened almond milk
• 1 tsp olive oil
• Salt and pepper to taste

Instructions:

1. In a small bowl, whisk together the egg whites and milk until well combined.

2. Heat the olive oil in a small non•stick skillet over medium heat.

3. Add the chopped spinach and sauté for 1•2 minutes until wilted.

4. Pour the egg white mixture into the skillet. Use a spatula to gently push the eggs from the edges into the center as they cook, tilting the pan to allow the uncooked egg to flow to the edges.

5. When the eggs are mostly set but still a bit wet on top, about 2•3 minutes, fold the omelette in half and slide it onto a plate.

6. Season with salt and pepper to taste.

This egg white and spinach omelette is an excellent choice for those following a no gallbladder diet. Egg whites are low in fat and cholesterol, while the spinach provides fiber, vitamins, and minerals. The small amount of milk or almond milk helps create a light, fluffy texture without adding too much fat. This omelette makes for a nutritious and easy•to•digest breakfast or light meal.

82. Baked tofu with sesame ginger sauce

Ingredient:

• 1 block (14 oz) extra•firm tofu, pressed and cut into 1•inch cubes
• 2 tbsp sesame oil
• 2 tbsp low•sodium soy sauce
• 1 tbsp rice vinegar
• 1 tbsp honey
• 1 tsp grated fresh ginger
• 1 tsp sesame seeds
• 1/4 tsp red pepper flakes (optional)
• Salt and pepper to taste

Instructions:

1. Preheat oven to 400°F. Line a baking sheet with parchment paper.

2. In a medium bowl, toss the tofu cubes with 1 tbsp of the sesame oil until well coated. Spread the tofu in a single layer on the prepared baking sheet.

3. Bake for 20•25 minutes, flipping halfway, until the tofu is golden brown and crispy on the outside.

4. In a small bowl, whisk together the remaining 1 tbsp sesame oil, soy sauce, rice vinegar, honey, grated ginger, sesame seeds, and red pepper flakes (if using). Season with salt and pepper.

5. Transfer the baked tofu to a serving dish and drizzle the sesame ginger sauce over the top. Toss gently to coat.

6. Serve warm, over steamed rice or with roasted vegetables.

This baked tofu dish is a great option for those following a no gallbladder diet. Tofu is low in fat and cholesterol, while the sesame ginger sauce provides flavor without being too heavy or greasy. The baking method also helps keep the dish light and easy to digest.

83. Mediterranean chickpea salad

Ingredient:

- 1 (15 oz) can chickpeas, rinsed and drained
- 1 cup cherry tomatoes, halved
- 1/2 cup diced cucumber
- 1/4 cup diced red onion
- 1/4 cup crumbled feta cheese (optional)
- 2 tbsp chopped fresh parsley
- 2 tbsp olive oil
- 1 tbsp lemon juice
- 1 tsp dried oregano
- Salt and pepper to taste

Instructions:

1. In a large bowl, combine the chickpeas, cherry tomatoes, cucumber, red onion, feta cheese (if using), and parsley.

2. In a small bowl, whisk together the olive oil, lemon juice, and dried oregano. Season with salt and pepper.

3. Pour the dressing over the chickpea salad and toss gently to coat.

4. Cover and refrigerate for at least 30 minutes to allow the flavors to meld.

5. Serve chilled or at room temperature.

This Mediterranean chickpea salad is a great option for those following a no gallbladder diet. Chickpeas are a good source of protein and fiber, while the vegetables provide vitamins, minerals, and antioxidants. The simple dressing of olive oil and lemon juice is easy to digest. The feta cheese is optional, but adds a nice tangy flavor if tolerated. This salad can be enjoyed as a main dish or a side.

84. Turkey meatloaf with mashed potatoes

Ingredient:

Meatloaf:
- 1 lb ground turkey
- 1 cup whole wheat breadcrumbs
- 1 egg, lightly beaten
- 1/2 cup low•fat milk
- 1 onion, finely chopped
- 2 cloves garlic, minced
- 2 tbsp tomato paste
- 1 tsp dried thyme
- Salt and pepper to taste

Mashed Potatoes:
- 2 lbs Yukon Gold potatoes, peeled and cut into 1•inch cubes
- 1/2 cup low•fat milk
- 2 tbsp unsalted butter
- Salt and pepper to taste

Instructions:

Meatloaf:
1. Preheat oven to 375°F. Lightly grease a 9x5•inch loaf pan.
2. In a large bowl, combine all the meatloaf ingredients until well mixed.
3. Transfer the mixture to the prepared loaf pan and shape into a loaf.
4. Bake for 50•60 minutes, until the internal temperature reaches 165°F.
5. Let rest for 10 minutes before slicing.

Mashed Potatoes:
1. Place the potato cubes in a large pot and cover with cold water. Bring to a boil.
2. Reduce heat and simmer for 15•20 minutes, until potatoes are very tender.
3. Drain the potatoes and return to the pot. Mash with a potato masher or ricer.
4. Stir in the milk and butter until smooth and creamy. Season with salt and pepper.

Serve the turkey meatloaf slices with the creamy mashed potatoes on the side.

This turkey meatloaf and mashed potato dish is a comforting and nutritious meal that is suitable for a no gallbladder diet. The turkey is a lean protein, while the potatoes provide complex carbohydrates and fiber. The simple preparation and ingredients make this an easy•to•digest option.

85. Grilled vegetables with balsamic glaze

Ingredient:

• 1 zucchini, sliced into 1/2•inch thick rounds
• 1 yellow squash, sliced into 1/2•inch thick rounds
• 1 red bell pepper, cut into 1•inch pieces
• 1 red onion, sliced into 1/2•inch thick rounds
• 2 tbsp olive oil
• Salt and pepper to taste

Balsamic Glaze:
• 1/2 cup balsamic vinegar
• 1 tbsp honey

Instructions:

1. Preheat grill or grill pan to medium•high heat.

2. In a large bowl, toss the sliced zucchini, squash, bell pepper, and onion with the olive oil. Season with salt and pepper.

3. Grill the vegetables for 8•10 minutes, flipping occasionally, until tender and lightly charred.

4. While the vegetables are grilling, make the balsamic glaze. In a small saucepan, combine the balsamic vinegar and honey. Bring to a simmer over medium heat and cook for 5•7 minutes, stirring occasionally, until the mixture has reduced by half and thickened slightly.

5. Transfer the grilled vegetables to a serving platter. Drizzle the balsamic glaze over the top.

6. Serve warm or at room temperature.

This grilled vegetable dish is a great option for those following a no gallbladder diet. The vegetables are high in fiber, vitamins, and minerals, while the balsamic glaze provides a sweet and tangy flavor without being too heavy or greasy. The simple preparation makes this a quick and easy side dish or light main course.

86. Chicken and vegetable stir•fry with rice noodles

Ingredient:

- 8 oz rice noodles
- 1 lb boneless, skinless chicken breasts, cut into 1•inch pieces
- 2 tbsp low•sodium soy sauce
- 1 tbsp rice vinegar
- 1 tsp sesame oil
- 1 tbsp olive oil
- 3 cloves garlic, minced
- 1 inch fresh ginger, peeled and grated
- 1 red bell pepper, sliced
- 1 cup broccoli florets
- 1 cup snow peas
- 2 green onions, sliced
- Salt and pepper to taste

Instructions:

1. Bring a large pot of water to a boil. Add the rice noodles and cook according to package instructions, about 5•7 minutes. Drain and set aside.

2. In a small bowl, combine the soy sauce, rice vinegar, and sesame oil. Set aside.

3. Heat the olive oil in a large skillet or wok over high heat. Add the chicken and stir•fry for 4•5 minutes until lightly browned.

4. Add the garlic and ginger and cook for 1 minute until fragrant.

5. Add the bell pepper, broccoli, and snow peas. Stir•fry for 3•4 minutes until vegetables are tender•crisp.

6. Add the cooked rice noodles and the soy sauce mixture. Toss everything together for 2•3 minutes until noodles are heated through.

7. Remove from heat and stir in the green onions. Season with salt and pepper to taste. Serve immediately.

This chicken and vegetable stir•fry with rice noodles is a great option for those following a no gallbladder diet. The lean protein from the chicken, fiber•rich vegetables, and gluten•free rice noodles make it a nutritious and easy•to•digest meal.

87. Baked halibut with lemon dill sauce

Ingredient:

• 4 (6 oz) halibut fillets
• 2 tbsp olive oil
• Salt and pepper to taste

Lemon Dill Sauce:
• 1/2 cup plain Greek yogurt
• 2 tbsp fresh lemon juice
• 1 tbsp chopped fresh dill
• 1 tsp Dijon mustard
• 1 clove garlic, minced
• Salt and pepper to taste

Instructions:

1. Preheat oven to 400°F. Line a baking sheet with parchment paper.

2. Place the halibut fillets on the prepared baking sheet. Brush the tops with 1 tbsp of the olive oil and season with salt and pepper.

3. Bake for 12•15 minutes, until the fish flakes easily with a fork.

4. While the fish is baking, make the lemon dill sauce. In a small bowl, whisk together the Greek yogurt, lemon juice, dill, Dijon mustard, garlic, and a pinch of salt and pepper.

5. Drizzle the remaining 1 tbsp of olive oil over the baked halibut fillets.

6. Serve the halibut warm, with the lemon dill sauce spooned over the top.

This baked halibut dish is an excellent choice for those following a no gallbladder diet. Halibut is a lean, mild•flavored fish that is easy to digest. The lemon dill sauce provides a bright, flavorful topping without being too heavy or rich. The simple preparation makes this a quick and healthy meal.

88. Quinoa and vegetable stuffed bell peppers

Ingredient:

• 4 bell peppers (any color), halved lengthwise and seeds removed
• 1 cup cooked quinoa
• 1 cup diced zucchini
• 1/2 cup diced onion
• 1/2 cup diced tomatoes
• 2 cloves garlic, minced
• 1 tsp dried oregano
• 1/4 cup crumbled feta cheese (optional)
• Salt and pepper to taste

Instructions:

1. Preheat oven to 375°F. Arrange the bell pepper halves in a baking dish or on a rimmed baking sheet.

2. In a medium bowl, combine the cooked quinoa, zucchini, onion, tomatoes, garlic, and oregano. Season with salt and pepper.

3. Spoon the quinoa mixture evenly into the bell pepper halves, packing it in gently.

4. If using, sprinkle the crumbled feta cheese over the top of the stuffed peppers.

5. Bake for 25•30 minutes, until the peppers are tender and the filling is hot.

6. Serve the stuffed peppers warm.

This quinoa and vegetable stuffed bell pepper dish is a great option for those following a no gallbladder diet. The quinoa provides a good source of protein and fiber, while the vegetables add vitamins, minerals, and antioxidants. The bell peppers are also easy to digest. The optional feta cheese adds a nice tangy flavor, but can be omitted if desired. This is a nutritious and flavorful meatless main dish.

89. Spinach and strawberry salad with grilled chicken

Ingredient:

Salad:
• 5 oz baby spinach
• 1 cup sliced fresh strawberries
• 1/4 cup sliced almonds
• 2 oz crumbled feta cheese (optional)

Grilled Chicken:
• 1 lb boneless, skinless chicken breasts
• 1 tbsp olive oil
• Salt and pepper to taste

Dressing:
• 2 tbsp balsamic vinegar
• 1 tbsp olive oil
• 1 tsp Dijon mustard
• 1 tsp honey
• Salt and pepper to taste

Instructions:
1. Preheat grill or grill pan to medium•high heat.

2. Brush the chicken breasts with 1 tbsp olive oil and season with salt and pepper.

3. Grill the chicken for 5•7 minutes per side, until cooked through. Let rest for 5 minutes, then slice or chop.

4. In a small bowl, whisk together the balsamic vinegar, 1 tbsp olive oil, Dijon mustard, and honey. Season with salt and pepper.

5. In a large salad bowl, combine the baby spinach, sliced strawberries, sliced almonds, and crumbled feta (if using).

6. Add the grilled chicken to the salad and drizzle the balsamic dressing over the top. Toss gently to coat. Serve immediately.

This spinach and strawberry salad with grilled chicken is a great option for those following a no gallbladder diet. The lean protein from the chicken, fiber•rich spinach and strawberries, and healthy fats from the almonds and olive oil make it a nutritious and easy•to•digest meal. The balsamic dressing provides flavor without being too heavy.

90. Turkey and vegetable soup

Ingredient:

• 1 lb ground turkey
• 1 tbsp olive oil
• 1 onion, diced
• 3 carrots, peeled and sliced
• 2 celery stalks, sliced
• 3 cloves garlic, minced
• 6 cups low•sodium chicken or vegetable broth
• 1 (15 oz) can diced tomatoes
• 1 cup frozen green beans
• 1 cup frozen peas
• 1 tsp dried thyme
• Salt and pepper to taste

Instructions:

1. In a large pot or Dutch oven, cook the ground turkey over medium•high heat, breaking it up with a wooden spoon, until browned, about 5•7 minutes. Transfer the cooked turkey to a plate and set aside.

2. In the same pot, heat the olive oil over medium heat. Add the onion, carrots, celery, and garlic. Sauté for 5•7 minutes until the vegetables start to soften.

3. Pour in the broth and add the diced tomatoes, green beans, peas, and thyme. Bring the soup to a boil.

4. Reduce heat to medium•low and let the soup simmer for 15•20 minutes, until the vegetables are tender.

5. Add the cooked ground turkey back to the pot and stir to combine.

6. Season the soup with salt and pepper to taste. Serve hot.

This turkey and vegetable soup is a great option for those following a no gallbladder diet. The lean ground turkey provides protein, while the vegetables add fiber, vitamins, and minerals. The simple broth•based soup is easy to digest. This hearty and nourishing soup can be enjoyed as a main course or a side.

91. Greek yogurt with pineapple and coconut

Ingredient:

• 1 cup plain Greek yogurt
• 1/2 cup diced fresh pineapple
• 2 tbsp unsweetened shredded coconut
• 1 tsp honey (optional)

Instructions:

1. In a medium bowl, combine the Greek yogurt, diced pineapple, and shredded coconut.

2. If desired, drizzle the honey over the top and gently stir to combine.

3. Serve chilled.

This Greek yogurt with pineapple and coconut is a great option for those following a no gallbladder diet. Here's why:

• Greek yogurt is high in protein and low in fat, making it easy to digest.

• Pineapple is a good source of fiber and contains an enzyme called bromelain that can aid digestion.

• Coconut provides healthy fats and a subtle sweetness without being too heavy.

• The honey is optional, as the pineapple and coconut provide natural sweetness.

This dish can be enjoyed as a healthy breakfast, snack, or light dessert. The combination of creamy yogurt, juicy pineapple, and toasted coconut creates a refreshing and satisfying treat that is gentle on the digestive system.

92. Baked eggplant with tomato and basil

Ingredient:

• 1 medium eggplant, sliced into 1/2•inch rounds
• 2 tbsp olive oil
• 1 cup diced tomatoes
• 2 cloves garlic, minced
• 1/4 cup chopped fresh basil
• 1/4 cup grated Parmesan cheese (optional)
• Salt and pepper to taste

Instructions:

1. Preheat oven to 400°F. Line a baking sheet with parchment paper.

2. Arrange the eggplant slices in a single layer on the prepared baking sheet. Brush the tops with 1 tbsp of the olive oil and season with salt and pepper.

3. Bake for 15•20 minutes, flipping halfway, until the eggplant is tender and lightly browned.

4. In a small bowl, combine the diced tomatoes, garlic, and remaining 1 tbsp olive oil. Season with salt and pepper.

5. Remove the baked eggplant from the oven and top each slice with a spoonful of the tomato mixture. Sprinkle the chopped basil over the top.

6. If using, sprinkle the grated Parmesan cheese over the eggplant.

7. Return the eggplant to the oven and bake for an additional 5•7 minutes, until the cheese is melted and the tomatoes are heated through.

8. Serve warm.

This baked eggplant dish is a great option for those following a no gallbladder diet. Eggplant is low in fat and easy to digest, while the tomatoes and basil provide vitamins, minerals, and antioxidants. The optional Parmesan cheese adds a nice flavor, but can be omitted for a dairy•free version. This is a simple and flavorful vegetarian meal or side dish.

93. Tofu and broccoli stir•fry with garlic sauce

Ingredient:

• 1 block (14 oz) extra•firm tofu, pressed and cut into 1•inch cubes
• 2 tbsp sesame oil, divided
• 3 cups broccoli florets
• 3 cloves garlic, minced
• 2 tbsp low•sodium soy sauce
• 1 tbsp rice vinegar
• 1 tsp honey
• 1/4 tsp red pepper flakes (optional)
• Salt and pepper to taste
• Cooked brown rice, for serving

Instructions:

1. In a large skillet or wok, heat 1 tbsp of the sesame oil over medium•high heat. Add the tofu cubes and cook for 5•7 minutes, turning occasionally, until lightly browned on all sides. Transfer the tofu to a plate and set aside.

2. In the same skillet, heat the remaining 1 tbsp sesame oil. Add the broccoli florets and stir•fry for 3•4 minutes until tender•crisp.

3. Add the minced garlic to the broccoli and cook for 1 minute until fragrant.

4. In a small bowl, whisk together the soy sauce, rice vinegar, honey, and red pepper flakes (if using).

5. Add the cooked tofu back to the skillet with the broccoli and garlic. Pour the soy sauce mixture over the top and toss everything together for 2•3 minutes until heated through.

6. Season with salt and pepper to taste.

7. Serve the tofu and broccoli stir•fry over cooked brown rice.

This tofu and broccoli stir•fry is a great option for those following a no gallbladder diet. Tofu is a lean, low•fat protein that is easy to digest, while the broccoli provides fiber, vitamins, and minerals. The simple garlic•soy sauce adds flavor without being too heavy or greasy. Serve this over whole grain brown rice for a complete and nutritious meal.

94. Chicken and vegetable kebabs with quinoa salad

Ingredient:

Kebabs:
• 1 lb boneless, skinless chicken breasts, cut into 1•inch cubes
• 1 red bell pepper, cut into 1•inch pieces
• 1 zucchini, cut into 1•inch pieces
• 1 red onion, cut into 1•inch pieces
• 2 tbsp olive oil
• Salt and pepper to taste

Quinoa Salad:
• 1 cup cooked quinoa
• 1 cup diced cucumber
• 1/2 cup diced tomatoes
• 1/4 cup chopped fresh parsley
• 2 tbsp lemon juice
• 1 tbsp olive oil
• Salt and pepper to taste

Instructions:

1. Preheat grill or grill pan to medium•high heat.

2. Thread the chicken, bell pepper, zucchini, and onion onto skewers, alternating the ingredients.

3. Brush the kebabs with the 2 tbsp olive oil and season with salt and pepper.

4. Grill the kebabs for 12•15 minutes, turning occasionally, until the chicken is cooked through and the vegetables are tender.

5. While the kebabs are grilling, prepare the quinoa salad. In a medium bowl, combine the cooked quinoa, diced cucumber, tomatoes, parsley, lemon juice, and 1 tbsp olive oil. Season with salt and pepper. Serve the grilled chicken and vegetable kebabs over the quinoa salad.

This chicken and vegetable kebab dish with a quinoa salad is a great option for those following a no gallbladder diet. The lean chicken and grilled vegetables are easy to digest, while the quinoa provides complex carbohydrates and fiber. The simple lemon dressing on the salad adds flavor without being too heavy. This is a well•balanced and nutritious meal.

95. Grilled shrimp with avocado salsa

Ingredient:

Shrimp:
• 1 lb large shrimp, peeled and deveined
• 1 tbsp olive oil
• 1 tsp chili powder
• Salt and pepper to taste

Avocado Salsa:
• 1 ripe avocado, diced
• 1/2 cup diced tomatoes
• 2 tbsp diced red onion
• 1 tbsp chopped fresh cilantro
• 1 tbsp lime juice
• 1 tsp olive oil
• Salt and pepper to taste

Instructions:

1. Preheat grill or grill pan to medium•high heat.

2. In a medium bowl, toss the shrimp with the 1 tbsp olive oil, chili powder, salt, and pepper until evenly coated.

3. Thread the shrimp onto skewers, leaving a little space between each one.

4. Grill the shrimp skewers for 2•3 minutes per side, until the shrimp are opaque and cooked through.

5. While the shrimp are grilling, make the avocado salsa. In a small bowl, gently mix together the diced avocado, tomatoes, red onion, cilantro, lime juice, and 1 tsp olive oil. Season with salt and pepper.

6. Serve the grilled shrimp warm, topped with the avocado salsa.

This grilled shrimp with avocado salsa is a great option for those following a no gallbladder diet. Shrimp is a lean protein that is easy to digest, while the avocado provides healthy fats and the salsa adds fiber, vitamins, and antioxidants. The simple preparation and flavors make this a light and refreshing meal.

96. Turkey burgers with lettuce wraps

Ingredient:

Burgers:
• 1 lb ground turkey
• 1/4 cup whole wheat breadcrumbs
• 1 egg, lightly beaten
• 2 tbsp diced onion
• 1 tsp Dijon mustard
• 1 tsp Worcestershire sauce
• Salt and pepper to taste

Lettuce Wraps:
• 8 large lettuce leaves (such as romaine or bibb)
• Sliced tomatoes
• Sliced avocado (optional)

Instructions:

1. In a large bowl, gently mix together the ground turkey, breadcrumbs, egg, onion, Dijon mustard, Worcestershire sauce, salt, and pepper until just combined. Be careful not to overmix.

2. Divide the turkey mixture into 4 equal portions and shape into patties, about 4•5 inches wide and 1/2 inch thick.

3. Preheat a grill or grill pan to medium•high heat. Cook the turkey burgers for 4•5 minutes per side, until cooked through and no longer pink in the center.

4. Place each cooked turkey burger on a lettuce leaf. Top with sliced tomatoes and avocado (if using).

5. Fold the lettuce leaf around the burger to create a wrap.

Serve the turkey burger lettuce wraps immediately.

These turkey burgers with lettuce wraps are a great option for those following a no gallbladder diet. Ground turkey is a lean protein that is easy to digest, while the lettuce leaves provide a low•carb,

97. Vegetable curry with chickpeas

Ingredient:

• 1 tbsp olive oil
• 1 onion, diced
• 3 cloves garlic, minced
• 1 tbsp grated fresh ginger
• 2 tsp curry powder
• 1 tsp ground cumin
• 1/2 tsp ground coriander
• 1/4 tsp cayenne pepper (optional)
• 1 (15 oz) can chickpeas, rinsed and drained
• 1 (14 oz) can diced tomatoes
• 1 cup low•sodium vegetable broth
• 1 medium zucchini, diced
• 1 cup cauliflower florets
• 1 cup frozen peas
• 1/4 cup chopped fresh cilantro
• Salt and pepper to taste
• Cooked brown rice, for serving

Instructions:

1. In a large skillet or Dutch oven, heat the olive oil over medium heat. Add the onion and sauté for 3•4 minutes until translucent.

2. Add the garlic and ginger and cook for 1 minute until fragrant.

3. Stir in the curry powder, cumin, coriander, and cayenne (if using). Cook for 1 minute to toast the spices.

4. Add the chickpeas, diced tomatoes, and vegetable broth. Bring the mixture to a simmer.

5. Add the zucchini, cauliflower, and frozen peas. Simmer for 10•15 minutes, until the vegetables are tender.

6. Remove from heat and stir in the chopped cilantro. Season with salt and pepper to taste. Serve the vegetable curry over cooked brown rice.

This vegetable curry with chickpeas is a great option for those following a no gallbladder diet. The chickpeas provide protein and fiber, while the vegetables add vitamins, minerals, and antioxidants. The aromatic spices add flavor without being too heavy or greasy. Serve this over whole grain brown rice for a complete and nourishing meal.

98. Baked cod with Mediterranean vegetables

Ingredient:

• 4 (6 oz) cod fillets
• 2 tbsp olive oil, divided
• 1 zucchini, sliced
• 1 yellow squash, sliced
• 1 red bell pepper, sliced
• 1 red onion, sliced
• 2 cloves garlic, minced
• 1 tsp dried oregano
• 1 tsp dried basil
• Salt and pepper to taste
• Lemon wedges, for serving

Instructions:

1. Preheat oven to 400°F. Lightly grease a baking sheet.

2. Place the cod fillets on the prepared baking sheet. Drizzle with 1 tbsp of the olive oil and season with salt and pepper.

3. In a large bowl, toss the sliced zucchini, squash, bell pepper, and onion with the remaining 1 tbsp olive oil, garlic, oregano, and basil. Season with salt and pepper.

4. Arrange the seasoned vegetables around the cod fillets on the baking sheet.

5. Bake for 18•22 minutes, until the cod is opaque and flakes easily with a fork and the vegetables are tender.

6. Serve the baked cod immediately, with the roasted Mediterranean vegetables on the side. Garnish with lemon wedges.

This baked cod with Mediterranean vegetables is a great option for those following a no gallbladder diet. Cod is a lean, mild•flavored fish that is easy to digest. The roasted vegetables provide fiber, vitamins, and antioxidants without being too heavy or greasy. The simple seasoning allows the natural flavors to shine through. This is a healthy and flavorful meal.

99. Quinoa salad with mango and black beans

Ingredient:

• 1 cup cooked quinoa, cooled
• 1 (15 oz) can black beans, rinsed and drained
• 1 mango, diced
• 1/2 cup diced red onion
• 1/4 cup chopped fresh cilantro
• 2 tbsp lime juice
• 1 tbsp olive oil
• 1/2 tsp ground cumin
• Salt and pepper to taste

Instructions:

1. In a large bowl, combine the cooked quinoa, black beans, diced mango, red onion, and chopped cilantro.

2. In a small bowl, whisk together the lime juice, olive oil, and ground cumin. Season with salt and pepper.

3. Pour the dressing over the quinoa salad and toss gently to coat.

4. Cover and refrigerate for at least 30 minutes to allow the flavors to meld.

5. Serve chilled or at room temperature.

This quinoa salad with mango and black beans is a great option for those following a no gallbladder diet. Quinoa is a gluten•free grain that is high in protein and fiber, while the black beans provide additional protein and fiber. The mango adds natural sweetness and vitamins, and the lime dressing provides a refreshing tang without being too heavy.

This salad can be enjoyed as a main dish or a side. It's a nutritious and easy•to•digest option that's perfect for warm weather.

100. Chicken and spinach stuffed bell peppers

Ingredient:

• 4 bell peppers, halved lengthwise and seeds removed
• 1 lb ground chicken
• 2 cups fresh spinach, chopped
• 1/2 cup cooked brown rice
• 1/4 cup diced onion
• 2 cloves garlic, minced
• 1 tsp dried oregano
• 1/4 cup grated Parmesan cheese (optional)
• Salt and pepper to taste

Instructions:

1. Preheat oven to 375°F. Arrange the bell pepper halves in a baking dish or on a rimmed baking sheet.

2. In a large skillet, cook the ground chicken over medium•high heat, breaking it up with a wooden spoon, until no longer pink, about 5•7 minutes. Drain any excess fat.

3. Add the chopped spinach, cooked brown rice, diced onion, garlic, and oregano to the skillet with the cooked chicken. Stir to combine and cook for 2•3 minutes until the spinach is wilted.

4. Spoon the chicken and spinach mixture evenly into the bell pepper halves, packing it in gently.

5. If using, sprinkle the grated Parmesan cheese over the top of the stuffed peppers.

6. Bake for 20•25 minutes, until the peppers are tender and the filling is hot.

7. Serve the stuffed peppers warm.

This chicken and spinach stuffed bell pepper dish is a great option for those following a no gallbladder diet. The lean ground chicken provides protein, while the spinach adds fiber, vitamins, and minerals. The bell peppers are easy to digest, and the optional Parmesan cheese adds a nice flavor without being too heavy. This is a nutritious and flavorful meal.

101. Pear and Walnut Salad

Ingredient:

• 5 oz mixed greens (such as spinach, arugula, or spring mix)
• 1 ripe pear, cored and sliced
• 1/4 cup chopped walnuts
• 2 tbsp crumbled feta cheese (optional)
• 2 tbsp balsamic vinegar
• 1 tbsp olive oil
• 1 tsp Dijon mustard
• 1 tsp honey
• Salt and pepper to taste

Instructions:

1. In a large salad bowl, combine the mixed greens, sliced pear, chopped walnuts, and crumbled feta cheese (if using).

2. In a small bowl, whisk together the balsamic vinegar, olive oil, Dijon mustard, and honey. Season with salt and pepper.

3. Drizzle the balsamic dressing over the salad and toss gently to coat.

4. Serve immediately.

This pear and walnut salad is a great option for those following a no gallbladder diet. Here's why:

• Mixed greens are high in fiber and low in fat, making them easy to digest.
• Pears are a good source of fiber and vitamins, and their natural sweetness pairs well with the walnuts.
• Walnuts provide healthy fats and a satisfying crunch.
• The optional feta cheese adds a tangy flavor, but can be omitted for a dairy•free version.
• The balsamic vinaigrette dressing is light and flavorful without being too heavy.

This salad makes for a refreshing and nutritious meal or side dish. The combination of flavors and textures creates a delicious and easy•to•digest option for those following a no gallbladder diet.

102. Egg Drop Soup

Ingredient:

• 4 cups low•sodium chicken or vegetable broth
• 2 eggs, lightly beaten
• 2 tbsp thinly sliced green onions
• 1 tsp sesame oil
• 1 tsp low•sodium soy sauce
• 1/4 tsp ground white pepper

Instructions:

1. In a medium saucepan, bring the broth to a gentle simmer over medium heat.

2. Slowly drizzle the beaten eggs into the simmering broth, stirring gently with a fork or chopsticks to create thin, wispy strands of egg.

3. Remove the pan from heat and stir in the sliced green onions, sesame oil, soy sauce, and white pepper.

4. Serve the egg drop soup hot.

This egg drop soup is a great option for those following a no gallbladder diet for a few reasons:

• The broth•based soup is easy to digest, as it's not heavy or greasy.

• Eggs are a lean protein that are gentle on the digestive system.

• The small amount of sesame oil and soy sauce adds flavor without being overpowering.

• The soup is low in fat and calories, making it a light and nourishing meal.

Egg drop soup is a simple, comforting dish that can be enjoyed as a starter or a light main course. The delicate egg strands and savory broth make it a soothing and satisfying option for those with gallbladder concerns.

103. Baked Halibut

Ingredient:

• 4 (6 oz) halibut fillets
• 2 tbsp olive oil
• 1 tsp lemon zest
• 2 tbsp lemon juice
• 2 cloves garlic, minced
• 1 tsp dried dill
• Salt and pepper to taste

Instructions:

1. Preheat oven to 400°F. Line a baking sheet with parchment paper.

2. Place the halibut fillets on the prepared baking sheet.

3. In a small bowl, whisk together the olive oil, lemon zest, lemon juice, garlic, and dried dill. Season with salt and pepper.

4. Drizzle the lemon•garlic mixture over the top of the halibut fillets, making sure to evenly coat them.

5. Bake for 12•15 minutes, until the fish flakes easily with a fork and is opaque throughout.

6. Serve the baked halibut immediately.

This baked halibut dish is an excellent choice for those following a no gallbladder diet. Here's why:

• Halibut is a lean, mild•flavored fish that is easy to digest.

• The simple lemon•garlic seasoning adds flavor without being too heavy or greasy.

• Baking the fish keeps it light and moist, without the need for frying or sautéing.

• Halibut is a good source of protein, vitamins, and minerals.

This recipe makes for a quick, healthy, and delicious meal. Serve the baked halibut with roasted vegetables or a fresh salad for a complete no gallbladder•friendly dinner.

104. Cucumber Gazpacho

Ingredient:

- 3 cups diced cucumber
- 1 cup diced tomatoes
- 1/2 cup diced red onion
- 2 cloves garlic, minced
- 2 tbsp olive oil
- 2 tbsp white wine vinegar
- 1 tbsp fresh lemon juice
- 1 tsp Dijon mustard
- 1/4 tsp ground cumin
- Salt and pepper to taste
- Chopped fresh herbs (such as parsley or basil) for garnish

Instructions:

1. In a blender or food processor, combine the diced cucumber, tomatoes, red onion, garlic, olive oil, white wine vinegar, lemon juice, Dijon mustard, and cumin. Blend until smooth.

2. Season the gazpacho with salt and pepper to taste.

3. Cover and refrigerate for at least 30 minutes to allow the flavors to meld.

4. Serve the chilled cucumber gazpacho garnished with chopped fresh herbs.

This cucumber gazpacho is an excellent choice for those following a no gallbladder diet for a few reasons:

- Cucumbers are high in water content and easy to digest.

- The raw vegetables provide fiber, vitamins, and antioxidants without being cooked.

- The simple vinaigrette dressing adds flavor without being heavy or greasy.

- Gazpacho is a refreshing, cold soup that is gentle on the digestive system.

This cucumber gazpacho makes for a light, nutritious, and flavorful starter or main course. The cool, creamy texture and bright flavors make it a perfect option for warm weather. Enjoy it as a healthy and easy•to•digest meal.

105. Stuffed Zucchini Boats

Ingredient:

• 4 medium zucchini, halved lengthwise
• 1 lb ground turkey
• 1/2 cup cooked quinoa
• 1/2 cup diced tomatoes
• 1/4 cup diced onion
• 2 cloves garlic, minced
• 1 tsp dried oregano
• 1/4 cup grated Parmesan cheese (optional)
• Salt and pepper to taste

Instructions:

1. Preheat oven to 375°F. Lightly grease a baking dish.

2. Using a spoon, scoop out the flesh from the center of each zucchini half, leaving about 1/4 inch of the zucchini shell. Finely chop the scooped out zucchini flesh.

3. In a skillet over medium heat, cook the ground turkey, breaking it up with a wooden spoon, until no longer pink, about 5•7 minutes. Drain any excess fat.

4. Add the chopped zucchini flesh, cooked quinoa, diced tomatoes, onion, garlic, and oregano to the skillet with the turkey. Stir to combine and cook for 2•3 minutes.

5. Spoon the turkey•vegetable mixture evenly into the zucchini boats, packing it in gently.

6. If using, sprinkle the grated Parmesan cheese over the top of the stuffed zucchini boats.

7. Place the stuffed zucchini boats in the prepared baking dish. Bake for 20•25 minutes, until the zucchini is tender and the filling is hot.

8. Serve the stuffed zucchini boats warm.

These stuffed zucchini boats are a great option for those following a no gallbladder diet. Zucchini is a low•fat, high•fiber vegetable that is easy to digest. The ground turkey provides lean protein, while the quinoa adds complex carbohydrates. The simple seasoning allows the natural flavors to shine through. This is a nutritious and flavorful meatless main dish or side.

106. Lentil and Vegetable Stir•Fry

Ingredient:

• 1 cup cooked brown or green lentils
• 2 tbsp sesame oil
• 1 cup sliced mushrooms
• 1 cup broccoli florets
• 1 red bell pepper, sliced
• 1 cup snow peas
• 2 cloves garlic, minced
• 1 tbsp low•sodium soy sauce
• 1 tsp rice vinegar
• 1 tsp honey
• Salt and pepper to taste
• Cooked brown rice, for serving

Instructions:

1. In a large skillet or wok, heat the sesame oil over medium•high heat.

2. Add the sliced mushrooms, broccoli florets, red bell pepper, and snow peas. Stir•fry for 4•5 minutes until the vegetables are tender•crisp.

3. Add the minced garlic and cook for 1 minute until fragrant.

4. Stir in the cooked lentils, soy sauce, rice vinegar, and honey. Toss everything together and cook for 2•3 minutes until heated through.

5. Season the stir•fry with salt and pepper to taste. Serve the lentil and vegetable stir•fry over cooked brown rice.

This lentil and vegetable stir•fry is a great option for those following a no gallbladder diet. Here's why:

• Lentils are a good source of plant•based protein and fiber, which are easy on the digestive system.
• The variety of vegetables provides a range of vitamins, minerals, and antioxidants.
• The simple sauce with soy sauce, vinegar, and honey adds flavor without being too heavy or greasy.
• Serving the stir•fry over whole grain brown rice makes it a complete and balanced meal.

This dish is nutritious, flavorful, and gentle on the digestive system • making it an excellent choice for those with gallbladder concerns.

107. Paprika Chicken

Ingredient:

- 4 boneless, skinless chicken breasts
- 2 tbsp olive oil
- 2 tsp smoked paprika
- 1 tsp garlic powder
- 1 tsp onion powder
- 1/2 tsp dried thyme
- Salt and pepper to taste
- Lemon wedges, for serving

Instructions:

1. Preheat oven to 400°F. Line a baking sheet with parchment paper.

2. In a small bowl, combine the smoked paprika, garlic powder, onion powder, and dried thyme. Season with salt and pepper.

3. Rub the spice mixture evenly over both sides of the chicken breasts.

4. Heat the olive oil in a large oven•safe skillet over medium•high heat.

5. Add the seasoned chicken breasts and sear for 2•3 minutes per side to get a nice golden•brown crust.

6. Transfer the skillet to the preheated oven and bake for 15•18 minutes, until the chicken is cooked through and reaches an internal temperature of 165°F. Serve the paprika chicken warm, with lemon wedges on the side.

This paprika chicken dish is a great option for those following a no gallbladder diet for a few reasons:

- Chicken is a lean protein that is easy to digest.
- The spices and herbs add flavor without being too heavy or greasy.
- Baking the chicken keeps it moist and tender without the need for frying.
- Lemon juice can help stimulate bile production, which is beneficial for those with gallbladder issues.

Serve this paprika chicken with roasted vegetables or a simple salad for a complete and gallbladder•friendly meal. The bold flavors and juicy texture make it a delicious and nutritious option.

108. Mushroom and Spinach Quiche

Ingredient:

- 1 pre•made pie crust (look for a gluten•free or low•fat option)
- 8 oz fresh mushrooms, sliced
- 5 oz fresh spinach, chopped
- 1 cup low•fat milk
- 3 large eggs
- 1/4 cup grated Parmesan cheese
- 1/4 tsp salt
- 1/4 tsp black pepper

Instructions:

1. Preheat oven to 375°F. Prepare the pie crust according to package instructions and place in a 9•inch pie plate.

2. In a skillet, sauté the mushrooms over medium heat until softened, about 5 minutes. Add the spinach and cook until wilted, about 2 more minutes.

3. In a medium bowl, whisk together the milk, eggs, Parmesan, salt, and pepper.

4. Spread the mushroom and spinach mixture evenly in the prepared pie crust. Pour the egg mixture over top.

5. Bake for 35•40 minutes, until the center is set. Allow to cool for 10 minutes before slicing and serving.

This quiche is a great option for those following a no gallbladder diet as it is low in fat and high in nutrients from the mushrooms and spinach. The milk and eggs provide protein without being too heavy on the digestive system.

109. Soy Ginger Beef

Ingredient:

- 1 lb lean beef sirloin, thinly sliced
- 2 tbsp low•sodium soy sauce
- 1 tbsp rice vinegar
- 1 tbsp grated fresh ginger
- 1 tsp sesame oil
- 1 tbsp cornstarch
- 2 cups broccoli florets
- 1 red bell pepper, sliced
- 2 cloves garlic, minced
- 1/4 cup low•sodium beef or chicken broth
- 2 cups cooked brown rice

Instructions:

1. In a medium bowl, combine the beef, soy sauce, rice vinegar, ginger, sesame oil, and cornstarch. Toss to coat the beef and let marinate for 15 minutes.

2. Heat a large skillet or wok over medium•high heat. Add the beef mixture and stir•fry for 2•3 minutes until the beef is lightly browned.

3. Add the broccoli, bell pepper, and garlic. Stir•fry for 3•4 minutes until the vegetables are tender•crisp.

4. Pour in the broth and bring to a simmer. Cook for 1•2 minutes until the sauce has thickened slightly.

5. Serve the soy ginger beef immediately over the cooked brown rice.

This dish is a great option for those following a no gallbladder diet as it is low in fat and high in lean protein, vegetables, and whole grains. The ginger and soy sauce provide lots of flavor without being too heavy on the digestive system.

110. Cauliflower Tabbouleh

Ingredient:

• 1 head of cauliflower, cut into florets
• 1 cup chopped fresh parsley
• 1/2 cup chopped fresh mint
• 1/2 cup chopped green onions
• 1/4 cup lemon juice
• 2 tbsp olive oil
• 1 tsp ground cumin
• 1/4 tsp salt
• 1/4 tsp black pepper

Instructions:

1. In a food processor, pulse the cauliflower florets until they are finely chopped and resemble the texture of cooked bulgur wheat. Transfer to a large bowl.

2. Add the chopped parsley, mint, and green onions to the bowl with the cauliflower.

3. In a small bowl, whisk together the lemon juice, olive oil, cumin, salt, and pepper.

4. Pour the dressing over the cauliflower mixture and toss gently to coat everything evenly.

5. Cover and refrigerate for at least 30 minutes to allow the flavors to meld.

6. Serve chilled or at room temperature.

This cauliflower tabbouleh is a great low•fat, low•cholesterol option for those following a no gallbladder diet. The cauliflower provides a similar texture to traditional tabbouleh, while the fresh herbs and lemon juice add lots of bright, fresh flavor. It's a healthy, fiber•rich side dish or light main course.

Adapting to life without a gallbladder can be a daunting experience, but with the right dietary choices, it is entirely possible to lead a healthy and fulfilling life. ***"No Gallbladder Diet Cookbook: Eating Well After Surgery"*** *has been your guide through this transition, providing you with the tools, knowledge, and recipes to navigate your new dietary landscape with confidence and ease.*

Over the past 100 days, you've explored a variety of delicious and nutritious recipes designed to support sensitive digestion and reduce inflammation. Each meal plan and recipe has been carefully curated to ensure that your body receives the essential nutrients it needs while minimizing discomfort and promoting optimal health.

The journey to recovery and maintaining a balanced diet without a gallbladder is a continuous one. As you move forward, remember to listen to your body and make adjustments as needed. The principles and recipes in this cookbook are here to support you, offering flexibility and variety to suit your evolving needs.

Thank you for allowing this book to be a part of your healing journey. May it continue to inspire you to make mindful and nourishing food choices every day. Here's to your health, happiness, and a future filled with delicious meals that support your well-being.

9 798328 791335